CHICKEN SOUP FOR THE SOUL IN MENOPAUSE

CHICKEN SOUP FOR THE SOUL IN MENOPAUSE

Living and Laughing Through Hot Flashes and Hormones

Jack Canfield
Mark Victor Hansen
Dahlynn McKowen

Health Communications, Inc.
Deerfield Beach, Florida

www.hcibooks.com
www.chickensoup.com

Hi Reta!

I Hope
you like
to laugh!

Ginger Kendall

Pg. 206-208

Dahlynn McKowen

We would like to acknowledge the many publishers and individuals for permission to reprint the following material. (Note: The stories that were written by Jack Canfield, Mark Victor Hansen, and Dahlynn McKowen are not included in this listing.)

Menopause Musings. Reprinted by permission of Lorraine Susan Mace. ©2006 Lorraine Susan Mace.

Changing. Reprinted by permission of Lisa L. Newkirk. ©2006 Lisa L. Newkirk.

The Menopause Blues. Reprinted by permission of Valerie Jeanne Palmer. ©1992 Valerie Jeanne Palmer.

Up a Tree. Reprinted by permission of Mary Jo Fullhart. ©2004 Mary Jo Fullhart.

(Continued on page 289)

Library of Congress Cataloging-in-Publication Data

Chicken soup for the soul in menopause : living and laughing through
hot flashes and hormones / [edited by] Jack Canfield, Mark Victor
Hansen, Dahlynn McKowen.
   p. cm.
  ISBN-13: 978-0-7573-0581-8 (trade paper)
  ISBN-10: 0-7573-0581-4 (trade paper)
  1. Menopause—Popular works. 2. Middle-aged women—Health
and hygiene—Popular works. 3. Menopause—Anecdotes. I. Canfield,
Jack, 1944- II. Hansen, Mark Victor. III. McKowen, Dahlynn.
RG186.C486 2007
618.1'75—dc22

          2007008967

Publisher: Health Communications, Inc.
       3201 S.W. 15th Street
       Deerfield Beach, FL 33442-8190

Cover design by Andrea Perrine Brower
Inside formatting by Dawn Von Strolley Grove

This book is lovingly dedicated
to the women of the world.
May you grow old gracefully,
enjoy life, and eat lots of chocolate.

Contents

2. FRINGE BENEFITS

3. IT'S TIME

4. YOU'RE NOT ALONE

5. IN THE NAME OF LOVE

6. A SECOND HELPING OF MENTAL-PAUSE

Menopause Musings

Who is this batty woman
with hormones all unstable,
who used to feel so confident,
but now is quite unable
to handle even simple tasks
with confidence and flair,
who cries and yells and rages
that life is so unfair?

Dear God, I think it's me.

Who is this dreadful woman,
who once was so delightful
to spend an hour or two with,
but now is just so frightful
that seconds seem like hours
and days turn into years,
who sobs and storms and threatens,
then covers you with tears?

Oh Lord, I fear it's me.

Who is this happy woman,
who thinks that life's a laugh,
whose confidence is huge,
there's no blockage in her path
to writing epic novels
at ten thousand words a day
with wild euphoric feelings
that she wishes could just stay?

Oh yes, that could be me.

Who is this frenzied woman
who's trying to contain
her mood swings and hot flushes,
which really are a pain?
So many times she's woken,
to find herself on fire,
with bedclothes drenched,
but feeling not one atom of desire.

Oh dear, I know it's me.

Who is this nutty woman
with her crazy sense of humor,
who terrifies her husband,
or is that just a rumor?
He's male and he should suffer,
we ladies know the cause.
Our monthly curse is followed
by the bloomin' menopause!

You've guessed, of course, it's me.

Lorraine Mace

Acknowledgments

We wish to express our heartfelt gratitude to the following people who helped make this book possible:

Our families, who have been chicken soup for our souls!

Jack's family: Inga, Travis, Riley, Christopher, Oran, and Kyle, for all their love and support.

Mark's family: Patty, Elisabeth, and Melanie Hansen, for once again sharing and lovingly supporting us in creating yet another book.

Dahlynn's family: Ken and kiddos Lahre, Shawn, and Jason, for their love and patience. Another book is completed, and now it's time to celebrate!

Our publisher, Peter Vegso, for his vision and commitment to bringing *Chicken Soup for the Soul* to the world.

Patty Aubery and Russ Kalmaski, for being there on every step of the journey, with love, laughter, and endless creativity.

Barbara Lomonaco, for nourishing us with truly wonderful stories and cartoons.

D'ette Corona and her amazing self—from coauthor liaison to friend, she does it all with great grace and true professionalism. Chicken Soup is lucky to have her as an integral part of the team!

Patty Hansen, for her thorough and competent handling

of the legal and licensing aspects of the Chicken Soup for the Soul books. You are magnificent at the challenge!

Veronica Romero, Teresa Collett, Robin Yerian, Jesse Ianniello, Lauren Edelstein, Lisa Williams, Laurie Hartman, Patti Clement, Meagan Romanello, Noelle Champagne, Jody Emme, Debbie Lefever, Michelle Adams, Dee Dee Romanello, Shanna Vieyra, and Gina Romanello, who support Jack's and Mark's businesses with skill and love.

Ken McKowen for his superb editing of the final manuscript. Thank you!

Michele Matriscini, Carol Rosenberg, Andrea Gold, Allison Janse, Katheline St. Fort, our editors at Health Communications, Inc., for their devotion to excellence.

Terry Burke, Tom Sand, Irena Xanthos, Lori Golden, Kelly Johnson Maragni, Karen Bailiff Ornstein, Randee Feldman, Patricia McConnell, Kim Weiss, Maria Dinoia, Paola Fernandez-Rana, and the marketing, sales, and PR departments at Health Communications, Inc., for doing such an incredible job supporting our books.

Tom Sand, Claude Choquette, and Luc Jutras, who manage year after year to get our books translated into thirty-six languages around the world.

The art department at Health Communications, Inc., for their talent, creativity, and unrelenting patience in producing book covers and inside designs that capture the essence of Chicken Soup: Larissa Hise Henoch, Lawna Patterson Oldfield, Andrea Perrine Brower, Anthony Clausi, and Dawn Von Strolley Grove.

Doreen Hess and the customer-support center and shipping department at Health Communications, Inc. Without all of you, the place would come to a grinding halt!

Shayla Seay for keeping our office humming along, taking care of all the small matters so we could concentrate on the big picture. Your loyalty and professionalism speak volumes about your dedication to this project. Thank you!

Our glorious panel of readers who helped us make the final selections and made invaluable suggestions on how to improve the book.

Our panel of readers who helped with the grading of the manuscript: Michele Caprario, Jackie Collins, Andrianne Cox, Rosa Dexheimer, Lisa Drutt, Jackie Flemming, Colleen Gannon, Lynne Haglund, Angela Hall, Julie Kaufman, Gail Kulhavy, C. J. Johnson, Scharre Johnson, Jennifer Martin, Cindi McKowen, Kathleen Partak, Joyce Rapier, Donna Rogers, Greg Seay, Shayla Seay, Diane Smith, Debbie Stack, Joanne Thompson, Teresa Tjaden, Aileen Van Noland, and Nancy Withers.

To everyone who submitted a story, we deeply appreciate your letting us into your lives and sharing your experiences with us. For those whose stories were not chosen for publication, we hope the stories you are about to enjoy convey what was in your hearts.

Because of the size of this project, we may have left out the names of some people who contributed along the way. If so, we are sorry, but please know that we really do appreciate you very much.

We are truly grateful and love you all!

Introduction

People like you and I, though mortal of course like everyone else, do not grow old no matter how long we live . . . [We] never cease to stand like curious children before the great mystery into which we were born.

Albert Einstein

Since I am the only female coauthor on this title, Jack and Mark agreed it was appropriate for me to pen the introduction. Smart men!

Creating this book has been different from the other titles I have produced with Jack and Mark, and for one primary reason: In reading the hundreds of stories submitted by people like you for this book, I had an epiphany—I was in menopause!

Prior to starting this book project, I was experiencing a great mystery in my life, just like the one Albert Einstein (one of my all-time favorites, next to Mark Twain) refers to in his quote above. Granted, you can interpret his quote in many ways, but I like to think that, as adults, we have the ability to retain a child-like exploration and curiosity about life. *I'll never get old,* I always happily said to myself.

Well, that fantasy came to a screeching halt in late 2005 when I had to hold a restaurant menu at arm's length! I was confused at first as I tried to focus, blaming my blurry eyesight on the fact that I had been working hard on the final manuscript for *Chicken Soup for the Entrepreneur's Soul.* I knew there was just no way that I could have problems with my eyes—I was the only one in my entire family who had perfect vision, and I teased my siblings and parents about it, a lot.

Then I started to get my kids' names mixed up. I called my teenage daughter Lahre by her younger brother's name, Shawn, and vice versa. *Huh?* They were just as confused, but more so when I started doing it more often, also calling them by their dogs' names—Shilo and Coco!

Next, my thought processes started to slip, and for the first time in my life I was at a loss for words. (If you know me, you're probably laughing because you know I can TALK!) I was giving a live, on-air radio interview for *Entrepreneur's Soul* from the comfort of my home office when I totally forgot the name of an entrepreneur from the book who started Famous Dave's restaurants. Again, the chain is called Famous *Dave's.* The answer is Dave Anderson, an amazing man and friend of mine. I stammered and stalled, then said, "Oh, we have many other wonderful entrepreneurs in the book," trying to steer the interview in another direction. When I hung up, I turned around and, lo and behold, on my desk was Dave's latest cookbook that he had sent as a gift. His smiling face and printed name were staring back at me.

By this time, Lahre and Shawn were onto my memory lapses and started with the, "Don't you remember, Mom . . . you said I could stay up past eleven?" or "Mom, you promised we'd have pizza tonight!" I would just stare at them, then look to my hubby Ken for back-up. His memory's worse than that of anyone I know, so he wasn't much help!

But the most upsetting thing was that I was hot (and not in the way Ken enjoyed most). I'm naturally cold due to my low blood pressure, but all of a sudden I was hot—really HOT—all of the time! And sweaty, too, and it wasn't only after my Jazzercise classes or treadmill workouts. *What in the world is wrong with me?* I worried, and often.

That's when I had my epiphany. I started reading all the wonderful stories sent in for this book—stories from vision problems and memory loss, to confusion and chin-hairs (I didn't want to share that personal story, but I do borrow Ken's electric razor every other day), to weight gain (another story I left out, on purpose) and hot flashes. Many of the stories mirrored my life *and* my maladies!

"Whoa, wait a minute," I proclaimed from my office chair one day when reading a menopause story about losing one's mind, "This is happening to me!" I startled my sister Shayla, who is our assistant extraordinaire. Never mind that she's nearly ten years younger than me and as beautiful and youthful as any thirty-something should be. She just laughed and said, "Lynnie, maybe you're starting menopause—you *are* in your forties!"

Menopause. The word hit me hard. Then I smiled, thinking of my childlike curiosity about life, my curiosity to explore new things and revel in new experiences. That's when I picked up the pile of submitted stories and read like crazy, learning from the women who have come before me. Thank you for your contributions to this book. I am forever grateful.

Dahlynn McKowen

Share with Us

We would love to hear your reactions to the stories in this book. Please let us know what your favorite stories were and how they affected you.

We also invite you to send us stories you would like to see published in future editions of *Chicken Soup for the Soul*. Please send submissions to: www.chickensoup.com.

Chicken Soup for the Soul
P.O. Box 30880
Santa Barbara, CA 93130
fax: 805-563-2945

We hope you enjoy reading this book as much as we enjoyed compiling, editing, and writing it.

Changing

Dimply thighs
Crinkled eyes
When did I grow this tummy?

Patience low
I just don't know
Why some think this is funny.

Can't lose weight
Running late
What is it I'm forgetting?

Money's tight
Don't sleep at night
I wish I could stop sweating!

Memory lapse
Strange need for naps
Some days I feel so lazy!

Happy, sad
Then raging mad
This "change" will drive me crazy!

Lisa Newkirk

The Menopause Blues

These menopausal sweats and shivers and shakes!
Lord, they're really more than a body can take!
One moment I am hot, and the next I feel cold,
Yet I'm told it's all to do with my "growing old!"

My teeth and my hair are departing from my head,
And my figure is developing that "hourglass" spread.
Wrinkles fast are multiplying all in a race,
To see which can be first to disfigure my face.

I need some new glasses to read the fine print,
And my joints squeal in protest if I have to do a sprint.
Although my needs are plenty and my pleasures are few,
My bones refuse to do what I tell them to do.

My heart palpitates at twice the given rate,
Yet when I need some energy, it's several beats late!
The very simplest chores have now become a huge task,
And if you want help, dear, please don't ask!

Sometimes I forget where I put things down,
Or even where I've parked the #$%& car downtown!
One day I am happy, but the next I'm full of tears,
And I often feel I haven't slept for seven hundred years!

To those lovely women out there who have aged with
    such grace,
Either someone's lying, or I'm quite a disgrace!
And to other ladies following, whose praises now I sing!
Ignore all the advice, and just do your own thing!

What was that you said, dear? I didn't quite hear,
But then, you know, I'm slightly deaf in my other ear.
In any case, please tell me, Lord, this won't last long,
Or these "menopause blues" could be my very last song!

Valerie J. Palmer

1

MENTAL-PAUSE

The most wasted day of all is that during which we have not laughed.

Sebastian R.N. Chamfort

Up a Tree

The best way to predict the future is to invent it.

Alan Kay

More than 50 million baby boomers turned 50 as the century came to an end. It's estimated that 35,000 women per day find themselves in the menopausal range. I am one of them. Growing up, I never heard the word "menopause." It was never discussed, or, if it was, it was whispered about in hushed tones between adults and behind closed doors.

When I began to suspect something funny was going on in my body, I went to the library to see if I could find anything on the subject. The good news was that I probably have one-third to one-half of my life ahead of me. The bad news was that I could spend a lot of that time having palpitations, hot flashes, night sweats, depression, loss of bladder control, roller coaster–like emotions, itchy and blotchy skin, insomnia, memory loss, urinary tract infections, and hair loss *and* hair growth in all the wrong places.

I slammed the book shut. When I began reading, I had all the above symptoms except depression. Now I was depressed, too! One thing I did find out was that heredity plays a large role when it comes to menopause. *My mother never had any problems, did she?* I thought to myself. I decided to call and find out. Our conversation went something like this:

"You know, Mom, I believe I am going through menopause."

I heard an audible gasp, then an "Oh, no."

"Mom, it's not a death sentence. Every woman goes through it sooner or later. You did, right? I know I was a teenager then and doing my own thing, but I don't recall. . . ."

"Oh, honey, honey. Don't you remember that summer I took your little brother and went to Kentucky on a bus?"

I was confused by her question. "Yeah, but what's that got to do with menopause?"

"Well, I don't remember why I went, and when I got there, I didn't know where I was. Your poor dad had to come and get us."

"What are you saying, Mom? I'm going to lose my mind?"

"Probably" was her answer, followed by a muffled sob.

"*Mother,* none of the books from the library says one thing about a woman losing her mind just because she's going through menopause. It actually can be a pretty smooth process."

I heard another sob. "Well, then, why are you asking me?"

"I'm asking you because family heredity plays a big role. I mean, you went through it fairly early, and so will I."

"Yes, but I went crazy," she said, and then blew her nose.

"*Mom,* you didn't go crazy!"

"Don't tell me I didn't go crazy. Do you remember after you were grown, you said you couldn't eat anyone's great northern beans but mine? They were always burned, that's why. You thought they were supposed to taste that way. Remember how shocked you were to find out home-made fudge wasn't supposed to be eaten with a spoon?" she explained. "I always meant to apologize to you kids for that."

"Mom, I always liked your beans and your fudge. The important thing is, you're not crazy now, are you?"

"I'm not sure. Your father says that's debatable."

Sweat popped out on my brow. "Okay, Mom, I tell you what, let's just drop it. Let's talk about Grandma. Did she do okay going through menopause?"

"Oh Mary, I wish you hadn't asked that."

"Why? What happened?" I heard more nose-blowing in the background. I braced myself for the worst.

"Honey, your grandma, God rest her soul, climbed a tree...."

I was glad that I was braced.

"... and she took off most of her clothes and ..."

My head was spinning. "Why did she take her clothes off?" I asked. "Don't tell me, she was crazy, right?"

"She went crazier than a loon. I think she got to sweating, no air-conditioning in those days, you know. We had the best breezes in those trees on the hill. Of course, later, she didn't remember doing it. It sure did embarrass your grandpa, though."

With all the strength I could muster, I said, "I'm sure it did. Well, Mom, I'm going to let you go. You've been very helpful. Tell Dad hi for me. I love you both."

"Love you too, honey. I'm so glad we can talk like this. Hope I helped. Bye-bye."

Just before hanging up, she told me to call her if there was anything she could do to help. I did ask one favor. "If you ever see me up in a tree, please call 911, and then ignore me." She was still laughing when we hung up!

A few weeks later, I was talking on the phone to one of our church's Sunday school teachers about my situation. She suggested I talk to my mother. I laughed until I cried, and then I shared the conversation I had had with her. She laughed until she cried, too.

Mary Jo Fullhart

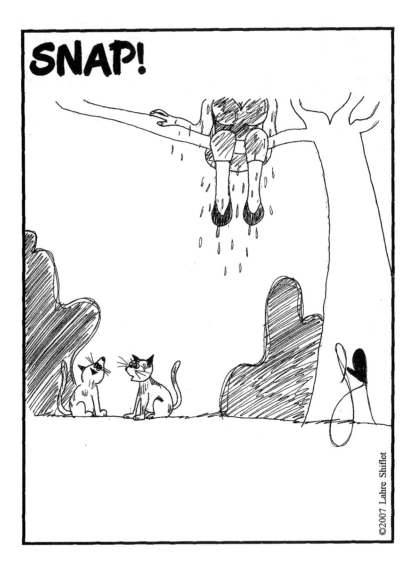

"You know, we could call the fire department . . . that's what she does when we're stuck in a tree."

I'm Melting!

"What are you doing in the freezer, Mama?"

"Cooling off."

Lisa laughed. "You look ridiculous!"

I pulled my head out of the freezer for a moment to study my daughter. "Who cares? At least I'm not disintegrating. You want to know what's ridiculous? I'll tell you. It's the dream I had last night. I was never more grateful to wake up in my life."

Lisa plopped down on the kitchen chair, with Bronwyn on her lap. Bronwyn is my two-year-old granddaughter. "So tell me."

"I was in a store, and the annual Christmas bash was only one hour away, when, all of a sudden, I felt a hot flash coming on!"

"Oh, no." Lisa was well informed on the woes of my menopause. She giggled.

"Oh, yes. Do you know what it feels like to have your body temperature rise a hundred degrees per second?"

"No. But I'm sure I'll find out someday."

"You can bank on that."

"So what did you do?" she asked, egging me on.

"At first, zilch," I replied. "My carefully applied makeup melted, and I had nothing left but raccoon eyes and a shiny face that looked like it was dipped in a vat of Crisco. And not only that, it felt like my scalp was burning and my hair had caught fire. Thankfully, a pool of sweat put the fire out. I panicked because I knew I wouldn't have time to reapply my makeup and go to the hairdresser for a fresh shampoo and blowout, let alone run to the boutique to buy a new silk suit before the party. You know how fragile silk is. So I did the only thing I could think of. I began to peel off my clothes."

"Good grief, Mama, you did *what*?"

"I began to peel off my clothes." Now I was the one who was laughing, along with Bronwyn. She loved my dramatics, a by-product of my spending so much time on the stage. "You should have seen the looks on the faces around me."

"I can imagine," Lisa said, totally scandalized.

"But it wasn't so much that I stripped myself naked that embarrassed me," I added, watching her horrified face turning interesting shades of red, "but rather the fact that I hadn't kept up my figure. There really was no excuse."

Lisa put her hands over Bronwyn's ears. Bronwyn smiled at me. She was a little nudist.

"The point," I said with all the unpredictable practicality of menopause, "is that I soon forgot my embarrassment in the blessed relief that I got from the store's air conditioning system. I could have stayed in that store all day. I seriously thought of not going to the party so I could do just that."

Lisa looked like she wanted to put her hands over her ears. But she couldn't. They were still on Bronwyn's. Bronwyn continued to smile at me. The darling, she was very comfortable in her skin, and if I didn't love her so much, I would've envied her.

"I cannot believe you did such a thing!" Lisa cried, appalled.

"Oh, for goodness sake, honey," I said, "It was just a dream." I shut the freezer door. I felt much better. But my hair felt crispy. "I need to buy more ice cream."

"It's at my house. You said you were on a diet and the best place to leave it was in *my* freezer."

The other thing that bothered me about mental pause, er . . . menopause . . . were my frequent memory lapses. "But Lisa, honey," I defended myself, "your house is thousands of miles away. Are you telling me I have to get on a plane in order to get some ice cream?"

"Well, you are watching your figure," she said reasonably. "You want to be skinny."

As if that's ever going to happen again in my lifetime, I thought. Oh, the sweet change of life—I wanted to rip its head off! Still, old dreams die hard. I still had my favorite skinny pants on a shelf where I could walk by them every day and salivate over them. I refused to give them up; I still fantasized I would wear them again someday, even if they were horribly out-of-date. Of course, Lisa wouldn't go anywhere I went when I wore them. But I was confident Bronwyn would. They would be back in style by then—for a teenager. Maybe we could go to the gym together.

Lisa looked at the travel brochures I had piled on the table. "Where are you going on vacation this year?" she asked.

"This year? Alaska. It's cold there. No beaches in the winter, no bikinis, lots of men. Did you know that men far outnumber women in Alaska?"

"You're married!" Again Lisa was horrified.

"I know!" I replied without batting an eyelash. "But do you realize how much good it does for an old broad's ego to think she can still elicit an admiring eye from the opposite sex, especially when she hasn't done anything to warrant it? That's a lot easier to do when she's bundled under a cloud of fur."

"You're impossible!" Lisa leapt up and, balancing Bronwyn on her hip, made for the freezer.

I stood aside, guardedly. "Just you wait; someday you'll be like me. In mental pause."

"Like you? Mama, I would never run around a store naked! Or go to Alaska to wink at men." Lisa stuck her head in the freezer. "I'm checking to make sure you don't have any ice cream in here."

The ice cream was hidden. Well hidden, behind all the diet items. Wisdom, albeit a sneaky sort of wisdom, is something else that Lisa would gain in time—besides weight when the estrogen receptors of the female brain are not supplied.

Janet Hall

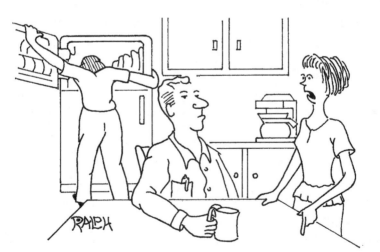

"She's *supposedly* looking for the fishsticks."

Feeling Better?

One Saturday, my husband of twenty-eight years looked pitifully at me and moaned, "I think I'm coming down with something."

"Why do you say that?" I asked.

"Because I have a scratchy throat, achy joints, and a little headache."

"Take some medicine, drink tons of water to flush out your system, and go rest," I advised.

"You sound like a doctor," he said with a slight grin. "So, where's some medicine?"

"Oh, brother," I rolled my eyes and snapped. "After all these years you don't know where I keep medicine?"

"I'm not feeling well. I don't want to think."

"Go look in the medicine cabinet or on our bedroom dresser."

The following Friday, we were eating breakfast in the wee hours before he left for work. "I'm still not feeling well," he sighed between bites of his cereal.

"I thought you were taking some medicine."

"I have been!"

"Well, what are you taking, sweetie?"

"Every morning, as soon as I get up, I take that medicine on the dresser."

"And you're still not feeling better?"

"I sleep like a log, but nothing else."

"Are you taking the right dosage?"

"It's dark when I get up. I don't want to turn on the light and wake you."

"Well, honey, read the box to make sure you're taking it right."

"I didn't see a box."

"There should be a box the medicine comes in."

"There's no box!"

"Medicine always comes in a box with instructions!"

"I'm just taking those white pills you laid out on the dresser."

"Which white pills?"

"The ones you have in a basket on the corner." We stared blankly at each other for a moment. Then his eyes narrowed and his forehead furrowed in thought. A smile broke out on my face.

"Those are my estrogen pills!"

Brenda Nixon

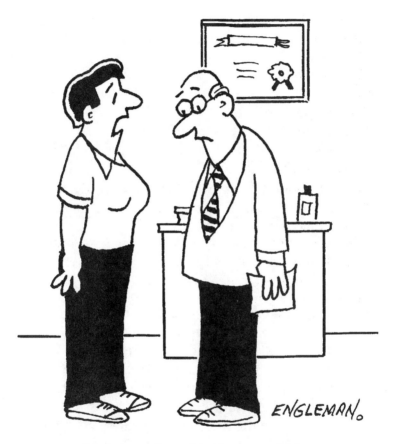

"Help me, Doc, I took several of
my wife's hormone pills by mistake!"

A New Routine

*The best and most beautiful things in the world
cannot be seen or even touched—they must be
felt with the heart.*

Helen Keller

For millennia women danced through life, preparing themselves to waltz, polka, or tango through menopause, that dreaded time when their brains and brawn were predicted to shrivel along with their reproductive organs. After centuries of fearing this dismal cycle, women began reading and overcame their fears by spreading the story in Genesis about Sarah and Abraham.

You remember the story, don't you? An angel of the Lord appeared to Abraham and predicted that his wife Sarah would produce a son. Standing behind their tent flap, ninety-year-old Sarah overheard the conversation and tittered with skepticism. Later, she fulfilled the prophecy and gave birth to Isaac (a record neither topped nor matched or recommended).

Nowadays, women accept this change-of-life period as just another challenge. By the time my turn arrived, I had one daughter in college, and I was still chauffeuring our other daughter—and her schoolmates—to endless high school and social events.

My first clue that I had begun menopause was my initiation into the sweating sorority. Yes, I know men sweat. Women perspire. But that doesn't apply during menopause. Like most inductees, I left my damp silhouette on my bedsheets every morning and carried boxes of tissues to absorb the rainforest seeping through my pores during the day. I quickly learned not to let my hormonal imbalance turn trivial incidents into emotional crises. And like all those women who preceded me, I persevered.

While living with the discomforts of menopause, I continued my motherly duties and endured noisy sleepovers, survived my daughter's driving lessons, and suffered sleep deprivation while awaiting that same daughter's safe arrival home from dates.

By now she was a senior, busy with extracurricular school activities, a part-time job and a driver's license. Suddenly, I realized that our television and stereo weren't constantly blaring, phones weren't constantly ringing, and my pantry and refrigerator weren't constantly raided. In this newfound peace, I resumed some of my favorite interests: music, sewing, reading, and writing.

One day while researching Middle Eastern cultures, I learned that belly dancing wasn't some wicked dance, but was a *danse du ventre* that dated back to biblical times. It was quite a revelation to discover that what I had regarded as erotic dancing was considered folk dancing in Mideast countries!

Hmmm... this could be interesting, I thought to myself. *The graceful arm and body movements might be an excellent way to firm my sagging muscles and redistribute my weight.* After more research, I decided that belly dancing might also be a good way to get rid of my stretch marks and shed some unwanted cellulite.

When I contacted our local parks and recreation department, the woman behind the counter snickered at my request. "In order to justify the expense of a teacher, you'll need to sign up at least twenty women." The haughty expression on her face and the smarmy tone of her voice left me feeling like she didn't think my idea was worth pursuing. Fortunately, my neighbors did. By day's end, I had the required signatures. I took my petition back to the recreation department.

Class information was circulated and sign-up lists for three classes were filled the same day. My glee turned to frustration when I discovered that my petitioners and I were put on a waiting list. After reminding the "snicker lady" that *I* was the one who had initiated the belly dance course, she relented.

Our full class listened attentively as our certified instructor gave us a detailed history of belly dancing. She taught and demonstrated body stretches, camel walk variations, scooting shimmies, head slides, and serpentine arm and torso movements.

She also played authentic Arabian music with delicate nuances of music moods that shifted between cheery, mournful, and lively melodies. Although the instruments had foreign names, we soon recognized flutes, zithers, drums, tambourines, mandolins, violins, and cymbals.

Among interesting facts she taught us was that in many Middle Eastern countries, belly dancers enter the delivery room and gyrate to music, encouraging the birth mother to perform rhythmic movements to promote faster and healthier deliveries. She emphasized that belly dancing wasn't a sleazy, sexy, cabaret dance, but a sensual dance filled with emotion that must be performed wearing proper belly dancer attire.

Hmmm . . . since I enjoy sewing, why not make a costume?

After buying a book illustrating traditional belly dancer

attire, I bought a blue two-piece bikini swimsuit and matching chiffon fabric. I also bought a CD of Arabian music that I played over and over on our stereo, memorizing the two-two and two-four beat while I sewed pearls and rhinestones onto the bodice, veil, and skirt band of my costume. Without telling my husband about my daring venture, I attended classes, practiced movements, and sewed while he was at work. By the time lessons ended, I managed to perform a fairly respectable routine.

Proof arrived several weeks later when my husband returned from an out-of-town business trip. He called from the airport, so I knew he was en route home, and thus I had time to set the scene.

We lived in a bi-level, so as soon as I heard our garage door grind open, I clicked on the stereo and positioned myself strategically at the top of the stairs. Wearing my costume, dangling earrings, and clinking bracelets and necklaces, I struck a sultry pose, flickered my eyelashes, and undulated with abdominal flutters to the exotic music.

By then, my husband was halfway up the stairs. He came to an abrupt stop, dropped his jaw and luggage, and grabbed the banister. After a quick recovery, he grinned from ear to ear and watched me perform traveling hip rolls, circles and thrusts, camel walk variations, head slides, and shoulder shimmies.

As soon as the music stopped, he dashed up the stairs, swept me into his arms, and whisked me off to our master bedroom.

When female friends question how I coped with menopause, I hesitate. *Hmm . . . should I share my story?* Then I confess, "Oh, I just followed the example of women who preceded us and danced to a new routine."

Sally Kelly-Engeman

Fuzzy Logic

If your ship doesn't come in, swim out to meet it.

Jonathan Winters

I was well prepared for menopause. I started reading up on the subject in my early forties. When it finally arrived sometime in my early fifties, I knew all about hot flashes, night sweats, and mood swings, which turned out to be annoying, but manageable, symptoms for me. More troublesome were issues of weight gain, aching joints, and a bladder that no longer held great quantities of liquids for hours at a time.

The worst symptom of all, however, was what I call fuzzy logic—that lapse between what the brain thinks is possible and what the body is able to do. I should have known better than to think my overweight menopausal body was in any condition to tear the roof off our garage the day I decided to do something nice for my husband.

Being a hopeless romantic, I delight in finding special ways to show my husband how much I love him, even after thirty-two years of marriage. I tuck love notes in his lunchbox, cook his favorite meals for no special reason, and plan an occasional romantic weekend rendezvous. This time, however, what he needed most was help with the garage roof since he had been especially busy with his electrical business. He planned to spend the weekend tearing off the old roof and putting on a new one. It would be a full weekend with no rest.

On Thursday evening, I spotted an odd-looking rake in the garage. "What's that thing?" I asked my husband.

"That's a rake for taking the old shingles off the roof."

"Oh."

Nothing more was said about the roof that evening, but I began plotting. *Wouldn't he be surprised and pleased if the roof was ready to lay new shingles when he came home on Friday?* I schemed to myself. I had the day off, and I was physically fit—well, at least I was at one time. This is where my fuzzy logic kicked in: *How hard could it be to take shingles off a roof?*

As soon as my husband left for work Friday morning, I slipped into my old Levis, slathered on sunscreen, donned a pair of leather gloves and a sunhat, grabbed a bottle of water, and slipped the cell phone into my pocket. Upon retrieving the shingle-rake from the garage, I looked for a ladder, but all I could find was a rickety old stepladder that had weathered too many seasons unprotected from the elements. *It would have to do.* Still determined to do this nice deed for my husband, I set the ladder near the back of the garage and started my ascent. It didn't reach all the way to the eaves, so standing on the very top rung, I hoisted myself onto the roof with great amounts of effort. I knew I would have to stay on the roof until I was finished because I wasn't going to try tackling that step again. *Better leave the water alone.*

I attacked the shingles with the all the gusto of my youth—for about an hour. Then my efforts slowed considerably. This was backbreaking work, and I wasn't as fit as I liked to think, but I was determined to finish the job.

Even catching the seat of my pants on a nail and ripping a large hole in them didn't stop me. There weren't any neighbors close by, so I just plodded away in my open-air britches. Between hot flashes and the warmth of the sun, my resolve to leave the water alone evaporated in the rising heat. *Surely my bladder could hold for a couple of hours.* Four hours later, when I pulled the last shingle loose, I was ready to collapse. I was also in dire need of using "the facilities." I gathered my things and inched toward the ladder.

The one thing I hadn't considered was getting back on that rickety ladder. I sat on the edge of the roof in a small state of panic. The ladder wasn't stable, and it was too far for me to reach the top rung without making the ladder sway. If I fell, I was going to have more than just a hole in my pants after landing on all those nails in the discarded roofing littering the ground below. I could only imagine what the emergency medical personnel would say upon finding a fifty-two-year-old woman with the seat of her pants ripped out lying in a pile of roofing material. That is, if I was even in any condition to call 911 after falling.

As I sat on the edge of the roof weighing my options, I didn't know if my need to use "the facilities" could overrule my fears of heights and falling. If not, I wondered how long it would take my husband to recover from his fit of laughter when he came home to find me stuck on the roof with a mysterious wet spot on the plywood. Of course, I could have called someone for help—if my menopausal brain had not forgotten that the battery in my cell phone was dead.

After nearly an hour of praying for enough courage to attempt a dismount, the call of nature was too strong to ignore any longer. I rolled onto my stomach and inched backward off the roof in the direction of the ladder, simply hoping not to break any bones when the ladder tumbled.

Thankfully, it didn't. But every muscle in my aching body reminded me that this venture was not one of my better ideas. After a hot shower and a couple of Tylenol, I returned the shingle-rake to the exact spot my husband left it and vowed not to say anything about my dilemma on the roof.

My husband was surprised and delighted when he came home to find the roof ready for new shingles. "How did you get up there?" he asked. "All of the tall ladders were on my work truck."

I pointed to the old stepladder.

He looked at the ladder and then at me. "I'm amazed you didn't fall. I've been meaning to throw that one away."

I didn't tell him that I was amazed as well. Sound logic would have made me think twice about ever climbing it. But since when do menopausal women have to be logical, especially concerning matters of love?

Caroleah Johnson

The Hormone Patch

This patch is doing wonders for my hormones.
At night I simply stick it on my tum.
One morning I was frantically searching,
Then I saw it there, stuck on his bum.

I tried to gently peel and not disturb him.
But firmly it was stuck, then he woke.
He jumped up late for work and started dressing,
Unaware of my own private joke.

Being late made him cranky and angry.
He snapped when I offered him food.
The door slammed, as I sat in my nightie,
Wondering if my patch would help his mood.

All day I couldn't help but giggle
As I thought of my patch in its place.
If only they could see through pinstripe,
That would sure put a smile on each face.

Pulling into the driveway, I was eager
To see how his day had turned out.

But instead of his usual greeting,
He started kicking his briefcase about.

He ranted his day had been awful!
And he thought that he must have the flu.
In the office he'd had twenty-seven hot flushes,
And tearfully ran to the loo.

His voice seemed a slight octave higher
As I sympathetically felt his head.
He announced to us all he had a migraine,
And in my slippers he flounced off to bed.

That night I removed the offending item.
I told the kids no longer to hide.
Tomorrow Dad would be back to normal;
He had just been in touch with his feminine side.

Louise Kelman

Menopause Strikes Fear

I hear and I forget.
I see and I remember.
I do and I understand.

Confucius

At the tender age of fifty, I was in my fifth year of hot flashes, hormonal highs and lows, and suffering from a general lack of patience with everything from traffic to my beloved cocker spaniel. I had opted to "ride it out" without the help of hormone replacement therapy.

For the hot flashes, I'd peel off clothing until I was often walking around the house in my underwear—it was impossible to wait until I'd reached the bedroom to disrobe because I was on fire. On the high swings, I found humor in everything. The lows would bring tears and woes. The Atlanta area traffic drove me close to road rage. At this point, my husband, who thought he ought to do *something* to improve life, suggested we sell our home in Atlanta and buy another with acreage in a less populated area of Georgia. We chose a neighborhood in the foothills of North Georgia, where all the houses had huge, heavily wooded lots. You had to work to find the driveways, and it was a long walk to all of the houses. It seemed the perfect place to "get Mama through this menopause stuff."

The first week in our new home was wonderful! The trees swayed in loud breezes, birds sang, and squirrels scampered noisily up and down the tree trunks. When I left the house, there were no traffic jams, no construction zones, and few fender benders to turn what should have been a five-minute trip to the grocery store into a five-hour venture. I could walk throughout the house bundled like a snowperson or in my birthday suit; there was no one to see me except God, my husband, and the dog. Then we were discovered.

Our first caller was a local minister inviting us to attend his church. He was clearly taken aback by my scant apparel and must have spread the word throughout the community because preachers and deacons from every denomination were ringing our doorbell three times a day by the end of the week.

Then the salesmen came. Every hour, our peace was interrupted by people who noticed we needed our grass cut, our pine straw replenished, our gutters cleaned, our windows washed. Men with trucks loaded with grandfather clocks came, and then others with refrigerated trucks selling meat came. There was no end—people started coming at sunup and were still selling late into the evening. We'd never had that many intrusions in our bustling Atlanta neighborhood, and worse yet, I had to stay fully clothed at all times.

Enough was enough! We installed a five-foot picket fence around the entire property, but it didn't slow the sales pitches down a bit. Then we placed a large "No Soliciting" sign at the gate to no avail. Next, we replaced the no soliciting sign with a huge "Warning, Guard Dog on Duty, Enter at Your Own Risk" sign. That one did slow the salesmen as they watched for a biting dog, but they still dashed for the safety of our front porch to ring the doorbell. "Lady," they'd say, "we just finished selling our clocks at the tradeshow and have a few left over. One of them would look good right over there," or "Ma'am, we've got an extra side of beef on the truck, and we'll sell it to you for a special price so we don't have to take it back to the plant" or "Miss, we don't think that church you're attending has a good plan for your afterlife." It went on and on!

Totally frustrated and desperate for the peace and quiet we longed for, I hastily hand-lettered another sign to post by the gate. It read, "CRANKY, MENOPAUSAL WOMAN ANSWERS DOORBELL!" No one came to the door.

Ah, menopause. Finally, a word that strikes fear in the hearts of all men!

Sherrin Newsome Willis

A to Z

Today is your day!
Your mountain is waiting.
So . . . get on your way.

Theodor Seuss Geisel (Dr. Seuss)

"That's it! You are now officially an outside dog!" I hollered, pushing my daughter's birthday poodle out the door. The pup had had yet another "accident," this time on my grandmother's quilt. I began sobbing hysterically as I tried to wash puppy poop from the quilt.

Looking up through a rainstorm of tears, I viewed the distorted faces of my daughter, son, and husband staring at me in disbelief. "And don't you dare let her back in!" I reprimanded. "I'm mad! You all insisted on getting this new puppy and nobody will feed or potty train her. Now I'm late to class!" I began my routine key and glasses search and five minutes later found my glasses on my head.

"Honey, are these your keys?" my husband meekly asked. "Somehow they got in the refrigerator."

Thank God it was Friday! After my last class, I headed

for a mountain retreat in Ruidoso, New Mexico. When I arrived at the cabin, Patsy, my teaching buddy, greeted me. Patsy and I were using this January weekend to plan our semester pen-pal program between her second-grade class and my college methods class. Thirty minutes into our planning session, Patsy doffed her clothing and made a beeline for the front door. "Patsy!" I cried out, "Are you crazy?"

"I'm flashing!" Patsy yelled from the front porch. I had been spared from the dreaded hot flashes thus far and had no idea they came on so abruptly. After Patsy returned and put on her housecoat, I laughed hysterically.

"Darn, you made me wet my pants!" I exclaimed. "Thank God I didn't sneeze. Then I'd need a diaper change!" We poured ourselves a couple of glasses of red wine and continued laughing and moaning about the stumbling blocks and pitfalls of menopause. Soon we began to create midlife limericks. After writing down a dozen silly limericks, it was decided at 2:00 AM that I would write a midlife alphabet book. Maybe humor was the medicine that would help me and my friends through this turbulent passage.

Three months later, my dream became reality. My limericks were in a book, complete with a clever colored cover and thirteen pen-and-ink cartoon illustrations. It was an immediate hit with my family and friends. I printed 100 copies at Office Max and decided I would perform a few at the Poetry Olio during the International Reading Association Conference in Indianapolis.

On the day of my trip, I packed my suitcase, slipping in twenty copies of my midlife book. Catching a plane in Albuquerque, I flew to Indianapolis, practicing my limericks the entire flight.

At the Olio, I was introduced by the host and was given five minutes to woo the audience. Drumming up my

courage, I said, "Wave your hand if you're a midlife girl!"
Over half the hands in the crowd of about 300 teachers
went flying into the air. "Great!" I exclaimed, "Then you
may relate to the limericks in my new book, *A to ProZac: An
Alphabet Book for Midlife Girls.*"

The crowd began to clap and laugh before I even recited
the first poem. "I'll begin with B." I continued, "B is for
Bladder:

> *I once had a bladder, you bet*
> *It ran like a fine-tuned Corvette*
> *Now pee leaks down my thigh*
> *When I laugh or I cry*
> *When I sneeze it streams like a jet.*"

The crowd roared and my confidence soared. "Thank
you, thank you very much!" I bellowed. "D is for . . ."

I paused to let the audience respond. "Depressed!"
someone shouted, followed by much laughter. Then
"diet!" someone else called out. "Yes!" I responded, "D is for
Diet:

> *I once could lose weight on a diet*
> *But now my body won't buy it*
> *The less fat I eats*
> *The more pounds I keeps*
> *So now I eat ice cream*
> *And FRY IT!*"

The audience broke out in laughter and wildly
applauded.

"Thank you!" I then prompted, "What is your guess for
M?"

"Menopause!" about a hundred women shouted at
once.

"That's a good guess," I agreed. "Think of something we
all have *during* menopause."

"Misery!" someone shouted, followed by lots of laughter. "Memory loss!" called out a few more voices.

"My M is for Mammogram," I said, and with exaggerated motions I recited:

> *I once had two breasts firm and fat*
> *Till thrown in that mammogram vat*
> *That maiming machine*
> *Pressed them real lean*
> *Now my breasts are a double A Flat!"*

Gut-wrenching laughter, "amens," and applause filled the entire room as I took my bow. "More, more!" they roared.

"Time's up!" chimed in the Olio host. "For the X-rated limericks, buy Karen's book!" I took my final bow, held up my book, and strutted offstage. But before I could collect my book bag and head to the "After Olio" celebration, I was stampeded by a herd of teachers. "Where can we buy your book?" ten of them shouted at once.

"Well, I have twenty with me." I replied. Then I looked up and realized that about 100 women were lined up for copies. "But I'll gladly take orders!" I quickly added.

Things were moving smoothly until I was autographing my next-to-the-last book. Two teachers were literally playing tug-of-war with the last *A to ProZac*. I looked at the one who appeared to be around twenty-five and questioned, "Sweetie, why would you need this book?"

"I need it for my mother," she uttered, eyes glassing over with tears. "She really could use a laugh. I want to give it to her this Sunday, for Mother's Day."

I looked at the midlife teacher competing for the book, and she now had tears in her eyes, too. Handing the book to the younger teacher, she said, "I know Mother's Day will be filled with love and much laughter for your mom."

"Thanks so much," I said to the older teacher. "Give me

your name and address, and I will send you an auto-graphed copy, on the house, as soon as I get back to New Mexico."

I took book orders from the remaining teachers and then headed to join the "After Olio" celebration with my favorite children's poets. I couldn't wait to revel in my success and perhaps even perform a few of the book's saucier midlife limericks!

Karen Alexander

What Amy Did

We all live under the same sky, but we don't all have the same horizon.

Konrad Adenauer

Some physical conditions are common to us all, no matter if you live in the United States or in Scotland, as I do. The difference is simply how we react to them.

The worst thing anyone ever said to my husband, Eric, was what his mate Davie said about his wife, Amy. Davie said, "Amy's fifty-four this year, six years older than your Joyce. Take it from me, Joyce will soon be at that *difficult age.*"

Naturally, Eric wanted to know more of what he was in for! Unfortunately, Amy, though I love her dearly, had every possible "difficult age" problem that existed, and she made the most of it!

To say that Eric is a forthright Scot just about sums him up. He asked me, "Am I in for all that hassle then, all those flushes and funny moods, bursting into tears all the time?" It didn't seem so much a question as a warning that he would not be at all amused if he was!

I just shrugged and said, "Who knows; it's nature. Not

much I can do about it if you are!" I retorted. The only downside to my retort was Eric's constant dread about when my "horrible" menopausal symptoms would start!

One night, I said to Eric that our bedroom was too warm. His reaction was immediate; since I'm nearly always cold, this set off his alarm bells.

"Davie said that Amy got some kind of tablets from the doctor that helped her!" was Eric's immediate response.

I just stared at him and asked, "What?" I sighed, realizing what he had said, and tried to keep calm. "I'm too warm because, as I have said before, the lowest tog duvet cover we have is much too high for warm weather. We have put in new central heating and double glazed the windows!"

Eric considered that and shrugged, "Well, yeah, I suppose that would contribute." Unfortunately, another one of Amy's problems was sudden dizzy spells. "She would be fine one minute and fainting the next!" Davie had explained to Eric.

One evening, I came in from visiting a friend. Just inside the living room door, I felt my head go round and steadied myself on the back of a chair. Eric got to his feet and offered, "Davie said that Amy used to put lavender oil in her bath and that helped."

I sat down and looked up at him, "Lavender oil for too much alcohol? Never heard that one!"

He studied me and repeated, "Too much drink?"

"I was visiting Lois and Mel, and he produced some of his homemade strawberry wine. It's blown my head off!" I confessed.

We went on for quite a few months like this. When I got on him about leaving shoes lying around, he got that look on his face, and I was sure he would tell me that "Amy drank dandelion wine from a bell pepper, when Davie left his shoes lying about."

Finally, I sat him down face-to-face and brought it all out into the open. "I am scared to just be myself because you are going to put it all down to the menopause. It's making me nervous!"

As we discussed it, I realized that Eric was scared, scared that I would change and he wouldn't know what to do. We managed to get it all sorted out eventually, but I did make Eric promise me one thing—that from then on he would stop listening to Davie and his tales of "What Amy did!"

I have to say that it worked. There was no comment whatsoever when a small tin of fruit was found in the hall cupboard and a small tin of paint in the refrigerator—mind you, that was because Eric put them there, not me!

Joyce Stark

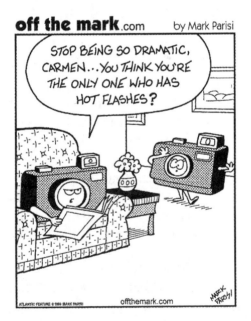

Reprinted by permission of Off the Mark and Mark Parisi. ©1999 Mark Parisi.

The Aztecs Are Coming!

It was the first time I had been out on the highway after Houston had made changes to some of their tollbooths. As we neared the tollbooth, my menopause vision took over.

"Well," I said, to my husband, who was driving, "that figures. These tollbooths have a separate lane to let certain people through for free."

My husband stared blankly ahead, his mouth open because, of course, the man was clueless as to what was on my mind.

"What are you talking about?" he asked.

"Well now, evidently we have Aztecs in Texas, and they are letting them through the tollbooth free."

I was greeted with a very blank look. He still didn't understand.

What is wrong with this man? I thought.

"Hun, what in the world are you talking about?"

I pointed to the last lane and said, "See, 'Aztecs.' They have a lane for Aztecs. When did that happen?"

He started laughing out loud. "That sign says "EZ

Tag."" He explained what it meant. I put my glasses on and laughed out loud, too.

To this day, my husband tells this story as often as he can. At least there is humor in menopause . . . sometimes.

Connie Parish

2

FRINGE BENEFITS

And this, too, shall pass.

Abraham Lincoln

Presto-Change-O

I'm still hot,
but now it comes in flashes,
I still got it, but to find it,
I'll need my glasses.

Alas, the pimples have subsided,
at least upon my face,
Now I have the finest of lines
to camouflage and erase.

Yes, I'm refining
like a quality wine
I only blow my cork
some of the time.

My figure may not be
what it once was,
Now there's much, much more
of me to love!

I'm wiser than
I was so long ago,
But, where are my car keys?
That's what I need to know!

Mother Nature may be cruel
and at times dreadfully unfair,
Tell me, why does she reward longevity
with gray roots and unwanted facial hair?

I'll get her back,
that nasty old hag,
For I have a few tricks
in my own makeup bag.

I have creams for dryness,
wrinkles, bumps, and spots,
And tonics to slosh down
when I get untimely *hots*,

I have many potions
to correct the gray,
And elixirs to vanish
that peach fuzz (ouch) away.

With a dab of this
and a pinch of that,
I tell you this
woman's looking PHAT!

Hurrah! Hurrah!
And yippee for me!
You see, I'm no longer
a hormonal-in-between,

I've graduated, and now I'm a
Many-Applause-al-Beauty Queen!

Jacqueline Michels

It Starts with an M

"Doctor," I said, "I keep forgetting things."

"Like what?"

"Ummmmm." What, indeed? There were dozens of examples, but suddenly I couldn't recall a single one. "Like all the examples I was going to tell you," I lamely finished.

"You're probably just under a lot of stress." *Yes*, I wanted to shout, *the stress of knowing that my mind is disintegrating, piece by itty bitty piece!*

Later, over coffee, my friend asked, "Why didn't you save yourself the doctor visit co-pay and just talk with me? I could have told you what stress you're under. It starts with the letter M."

"Memory loss?"

"Here's another clue: You could call it estrogen withdrawal."

"Oh, menopause," I said. "Well, at least it isn't Alzheimer's. Does this mean you've been forgetting things, too?"

"Let's just say that I don't enjoy watching *Jeopardy* as much as I used to," my friend responded.

Her comment made me smile. I should probably come out of the closet now and confess that when I was in high school, I was on the *It's Academic* team, a local television quiz show in which area schools competed every week.

I used to know all sorts of trivia, from the countries and capitals of Africa (my favorite was Ouagadougou, in Upper Volta, now Burkina Faso), to who wrote the song "Baubles, Bangles and Beads," to who ran against Harry S Truman in his second campaign for President (trick question—*he ran only once*). Plus, for extra credit, there should not be a dot after the S in his name, as he always insisted it doesn't stand for anything.

Nowadays, I'm lucky if I remember my own middle name. Too often, I find myself staring into the refrigerator, not seeing whatever I was looking for because I couldn't remember what it was, only to close the refrigerator and go back to whichever room I had come from, sit down again, and remember: "Oh, yes, a cup of coffee!" Repeat that process a dozen times a day and then wonder where the time has gone.

Another thing I never remember is where I left my glasses. Every night and every morning my children must help in the search, because I refuse to wear the librarian-strings people give me. "As lost as Mommy's glasses," my son once contributed as an example of "simile" in English class.

Worst of all for a compulsive talker and writer, I have begun to find myself at a loss for words. "I know it begins with a K," I said when my younger child asked me for another word for "curdle." Six days later, I was driving the older one somewhere when it finally came to me: "coagulate!" Well, at least it sounds like a K.

I wonder if we could design a new game show for me. Let's call it "Menopausal Pursuit" or "Menopause Jeopardy!" Categories could be "Names," "Places," "Objects," "Faces," and "Data," all followed by the phrase, " . . . that I used to know."

For example: When you run into someone who "looks familiar," do you at least remember having met them before? Good! Ten points! Do you remember where? Fifty points! Never mind their name—they probably don't remember yours, either.

When your answer to a question is "I don't remember the word, but I know it starts with an 'S'," you get fifty points. Or when a child picks up a knick-knack in your house, twenty points if you can remember where (or who) you got it from before it hits the ground.

And instead of Double Jeopardy when you pick the secret square, you will be randomly overcome with sudden hot flashes. And, in the Final Round, no one has to bother with the actual answer. Instead, full credit will be awarded to every contestant who leaps up after the answer is revealed and shouts out "I knew that!"

The prize will be a pad of paper and a pencil for writing down whatever it is you were looking for in the refrigerator. Just don't put down "my mind." That's gone forever.

Judy Epstein

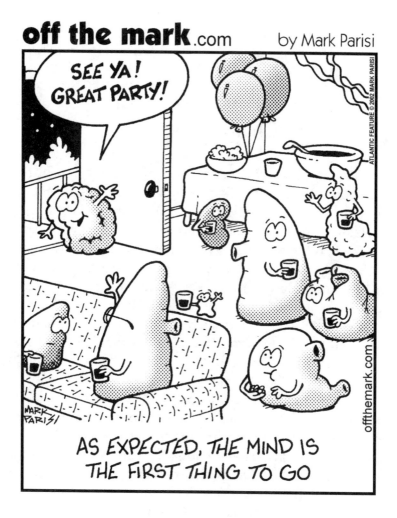

Chinny Chin Chin

I started menopause early, just after forty. I'm in that one-percent category. Okay, so I'm a statistic, every statistic. I've got it all, vasomotor instability, urogenital atrophy, skeletal twingeritus, soft tissue issues, and psychological sways. In other words, I have flashes so hot I have to rip my clothes off in public. I haven't slept in six years. I'm as dry as the Sahara Desert, and if I scratch my rashes anymore, I'll look like a boneless breast of chicken. Then there's the need to pee—a lot. There's muscle pain, back pain, and phantom pain. And just when you think it's not that bad, wrinkles, mood disturbance, irritability, fatigue, decreased libido, and, oh, before I forget, memory loss.

Did I mention whiskers? I handled everything else with below-average decorum, but I needed cognitive therapy for the whiskers. They were the last straw. Actually, they are the last straw. They're so stiff I can sweep the patio floor with my chin. And whiskers don't exactly fit with my image of femininity. My son concurs and tells me I'm metamorphosing into a man. I explained to him that whiskers are something that happens to old ladies, and that one day he too would age, but worse still, he'd grow boobs.

"Why don't you just donate all those chin whiskers to

science, Mom?" he asked. "Maybe they can transplant them onto a bald man or something."

"How about you run off and play with that bully next door, like a good boy," I barked.

"You can always ask Dad for shaving lessons!" he shouted, getting in the last word and narrowly dodging a bottle of airborne Nair.

There's a hardy, brawny whisker on the lower right part of my chin—it was my first. I didn't notice it until a friend pointed it out at a wedding. She went to pick it off me, but it uncoiled itself and strangled her. Bless her heart, and may she rest in peace.

Sadly, though, I'm actually starting to look like my wiry terrier Grace. The other day at the park, a Great Dane mistook me for her. It'll take forever to get that urine stain off my cream silk pants.

This whole menopause thing is an outrage. No one adequately prepares us for menopause. If they do, it's lies, all lies. When I exhibited the first milder symptoms, my doctor assured me that everything would be okay, and that in fact, I'd entered into the "climacteric" period of perimenopause, the stage just before actual menopause. Wow—talk about anticipation! Excited, I raced home to tell my husband. He got excited too, and for once, the crop of growth on my chin didn't make him vomit. We tried and tried, but never reached that explosive peak the doctor promised.

She also said that the hormone levels in my body would fluctuate and cause changes similar to the changes associated with an adolescent. Well, that got my husband excited all over again thinking I would metamorphose into Britney Spears. I did, sort of, with the help of Blonde Bombshell #59 to cover the gray. But there was nothing I could do to perk up my boobs. Then there were the hot flashes. Combine those with whiskers, and it's a recipe for prickly heat, I tell you.

You may think I'm obsessed with my looks, but I'm not. I just don't want to look like a nanny goat. Woe is he who makes any mention of bearded ladies, porcupines, or gorillas within earshot of me.

There's a saying out there, and that is: "Pull a whisker from a cat, get a claw mark on your back. Pull a whisker from a man, turn and run as fast as you can. Pull a whisker from your wife, pray to God there's an afterlife."

I know I can't take my tweezers with me when I die, but I'm going to ask God anyhow.

Shae Cooke

Best or Better

*You can complain because roses have thorns,
or you can rejoice because thorns have roses.*

Tom Wilson, Ziggy

I have a great idea for an invention. Inexpensive to manufacture, it would help millions of forty-somethings in denial. If designed correctly, the "Extend-o-Arm" would snap comfortably on to your wrist in a matter of seconds. With your arm length extended to forty-five feet, there wouldn't be a need to hear your optometrist say the dreaded words, "It's time to consider reading glasses."

Who ever dreamed we'd be in this predicament? First, all the estrogen was sucked out of our bodies by some mysterious force. If that wasn't bad enough, now we can't read the label of our hormone replacement medication. "I think it says to take it three times a day for the rest of my life," I said to my forty-something husband one morning. I handed him the bottle. "Can you read it?" He took off his non-bifocal glasses and propped the medicine bottle on his nose. His eyes crossed.

"It says take once a day!" he gasped.

"Uh-oh," I replied, "I'm sure there's minimal long-term damage."

He grimaced. "I didn't want to say anything, honey, but lately I've been noticing a three o'clock shadow on your face at nine o'clock in the morning." We left immediately to shop for reading glasses.

My husband and I stood in front of the display at the local discount store. "Look at the variety!" my husband said loudly.

"Ssssh!" I hissed. "I don't want to draw attention to the fact that I am in the senior citizen section of the store!" I had an image to keep up, for goodness' sake. The blind forty-something in denial image was not an easy one to maintain, but I'd been doing a pretty good job so far.

"Do you realize that in just a few years we'll be eligible for a senior citizen discount and the early bird specials at Joe's Diner?" my husband mentioned. I knew there was some good reason why I had married him—I just couldn't think of it at that moment.

I looked at the glasses on display. There were unrecognizable numbers on the lenses. "What's the difference between 1.00 and 2.00?" I asked.

"Try a 2.00 pair," my husband urged. "Bigger always means better." I put on a pair of glasses trimmed in a leopard print and looked in the tiny, blurry mirror attached to the display. My grandma stared back at me. I turned to look at my husband. His face contorted in fear.

"Your eyes look HUGE!" he said. "You look like Marty Feldman in the movie *Young Frankenstein!*"

This was not going well, but I had to face reality. I could no longer have the grocery store checker hold my checkbook in front of her so I could see to write the amount. And the Extend-o-Arm would take years to patent and manufacture.

After much browsing, I finally decided on a pair that

folded up into the size of a quarter. I figured the compactness of the glasses would be easy to hide in my hand, just in case I ran into one of my other forty-something friends and had to quickly rip the glasses off my face in order to maintain my image.

"Shall we buy the chain to go with the glasses?" my husband asked.

"Unless you want me to wrap that chain around your neck, I suggest you never mention reading-glass chains again."

Later at home, I picked up a book and put on my reading glasses. "My goodness!" I yelled.

My husband came running. "What is it?" he asked.

I pulled down my reading glasses and looked at him over them (I could do cool things like that now). "I CAN READ! It's a miracle!" I hated to admit it, but the words were clear, dark and, well—legible.

"I think I like you in your new glasses, my little Marty Feldman Jr.," my husband said lovingly. Just like we managed to get used to my estrogen-less body, I figured we'd both get used to these reading glasses.

And maybe, just maybe, the reading glasses would keep me out of the large print section at the library, at least for another year.

Vicky DeCoster

A Time to Remember

*Our memories are card indexes consulted and
then returned in disorder by authorities whom
we do not control.*

Cyril Connolly

"Do you sell sand?" I asked the cashier at the home
store.

"What kind are you looking for?" she asked.

"The kind you put in a sand . . . oh, jeez, what's it called
. . . the square plaything?" For the fourteenth time that day
I couldn't think of the word I needed.

"Sandbox?" she asked, looking at me sympathetically.
Good Lord, I thought. *I just used the first half of the word and
still couldn't think of it.* She obviously had children and was
over forty, or the sympathy look would have been more of
a lady-are-you-okay? look. Believe me, I know the difference. I've gotten them both enough times lately.

I honestly don't know what's going on here. I mean,
sure, I've done all the reading about pre-menopausal brain
fog and the memory issues associated with aging, but it's
all made to sound so benign, amusing even. Well, let me

say this to the powers that be, whoever you are: I am not amused. My husband might be, but I am not.

I used to think it was funny, I'll admit. I'd joke about how some people forget their grocery lists, while I forget to go to the store. But we're beyond that sophomoric humor, my friends. I am now writing notes in the bathroom to remind me to look at a note in the bedroom which reminds me to add something to my grocery list in the kitchen. It's like one of those strings people use to follow an unfamiliar path, or the ropes that are used in mountain climbing so that people can find the trail back down. My rope, sadly, is used to retain a thought.

Need more? I came out of the mall recently after having had lunch—lunch, not an all-day shopping spree—and I couldn't remember where I parked the car. And it wasn't the cute, "Oh, silly me, I'm in the next row over," it was, "Oh my God, someone stole my car! Wait—what was in my car? Garbage? Who'd want to steal my garbage?" As I stood there mulling this over, a kindly young man approached and timidly asked, "Um, can I help you find your car?"

He spoke to me as if I were ninety. And when I'm ninety, maybe I will graciously accept the offer. But I'm not ninety, I'm forty-four. "No, you may not," I snapped. "I'm perfectly capable of finding my own car." And I did . . . thirty minutes later.

At least that was a more or less private humiliation. The public ones are not as easy to sweep under the rug, assuming I'd even remember to get out the broom. These include the requisite forgotten appointments, birthdays, and anniversaries. They also include the time I invited people to play golf and then forgot to show up.

In that same vein, I invited my in-laws over for dinner on my golfing league night. It's been on Monday nights for three months, and yet I called and said, "Want to come over for a cookout on Monday night?" I told my husband later that day, and he gently suggested that it's probably bad form to invite your in-laws to dinner when you won't actually be home.

My kids think it's a riot, this memory issue, and have figured out how to turn it to their advantage.

"Mom, don't you remember last time telling me I could have this toy the next time we came here?"

"Mom, I asked you if I could have a sleepover with fifteen friends and you said yes. You just don't remember."

"Don't you remember that you said we could go to Disney World this summer?"

So I'm taking control. I bought some super-powered "scientifically proven" herbal supplements that are supposed to go directly to the part of the brain that's misfiring and improve, specifically, short-term memory. There are studies that show how this works. It's all very technical and medicinal-sounding. Unfortunately I have no idea if they work for me or not . . . I can't remember to take them.

Maggie Lamond Simone

A Little Blurry, That's All

The more sand that has escaped from the hour-glass of our life, the clearer we should see through it.

Jean Paul

There wasn't a dramatic difference from one day to another. Like a well-loved sweater or teddy bear showing its age, life had just become fuzzier. My usual eagle-eye vision had been replaced by squinting at street signs. Not that it matters, for in the small village where I live, I pretty much know my way around blind. I had no problem reading books or doing needlework, so I thought it must be allergies.

The lake road is my favorite place to walk with my dog, full of whispering pines and weaving roadways. It's home to eagles and beagles, horses and hares, also the odd black bear and other critters that are a bit grumpy if you come within sight of them. So it was no surprise one day when I stopped dead in my tracks, sure that the black thing several paces away was a large black bear. I reached for the bear repellant, prepared to do battle, and started banging my stick and yelling to scare it away. My dog was a bit stunned by my reaction and pulled me on to what turned out was an abandoned tire by the roadside. So as not to hurt my feelings, she gave it a good "ruff."

Luckily, dogs don't talk; they keep the best secrets. I was sure that it was just a momentary thing, after all I was just forty-two and the only one in my family whose eyes were 20/20, something I was always quite proud of! I had problems only in the evening when my eyes were tired; after all, I had used them all day. So while watching a foreign film one evening, I was surprised that I could not read the movie subtitles. I asked my glass-clad lad of a husband to read them for me.

He put his paper down and sounding very tired, he read the following from the screen: "Greta says, 'I love you, my handsome young cad, but what about Roland?' Hans says, 'Roland is a wimp and shall never hold a candle to me.' 'Never mind, Princess Leah, I shall defend you and the force with my highly attuned sight and intellect.' Greta says, 'But is that not Roland sneaking up behind you?' Hans says, 'Oh my love, my love, my love, I have been outdone by a don with spectacles.'"

My husband collapsed in laughter while I moved my chair closer to the screen to find out what the real dialogue was. It was then that I decided it was probably time to have my eyes checked. I made an appointment.

At my appointment, I sat in a darkened room and read from the large chart on the wall while the doctor made sure I didn't peek or cheat. He then put drops in my eyes, which made me look like some deranged cartoon character with pupils as big as saucers. As he checked for problems deep within my eyes, I reflected on how glasses would change my life. *Was I really ready for this?* I thought. *Am I admitting I'm growing old?*

Off to the eyeglass shop with prescription in hand, I

was thrilled to see glasses with titanium frames, Elton John frames, even the latest country look in rhinestones. There were frame colors that could bring out the highlights in my once clear eyes, sexy glasses, nerdy glasses, and even glasses to make you look smarter. I settled on those.

I tried on the glasses for the first time at home, sitting on the porch. The green of the leaves that had once looked like a moss-covered blanket now took on individual seams and sheens of green, gold, and jade. Every blade of grass stood up, unique and sharp as quills. Even the hair on the dog, that used to blend together, showed lustrous individual hairs of black, brown, and silver. I was in awe.

I have discovered that I am not blind to the latest fashion. Just as my daughter, who is years before me in the eye department, seeks out the latest music, I do my own shopping. As my excited voice filters from the mall's eyeglass shop into the nearby CD shop, customers look up and wonder who that woman is raving about frames and gadgets and glass cases.

"Don't worry," my contact-wearing daughter sighs to the salesclerk, "it's only my mom, making a spectacle of herself again."

Nancy Bennett

Go with the Flow

*When I have to choose between two evils, I
always try to pick the one I haven't tried before.*

Mae West

Menopause hit me fast; everything I ate automatically
went to my waist, my mood swings sadistically pushed
me to see how high I could fly, and the night sweats began
at dusk and ended the next day at 5:59 AM. No wonder
other symptoms came on with such a vengeance, like my
memorable moment at the grocery store after a mega-
emotional day at work.

As was habit, I obeyed the sign to "start with a cart."
With shopping list in hand, arranged in my usual path
through the store, I dashed off, hopeful to complete my
appointed course without having to wait too long at
checkout.

Please, God! I thought to myself, *Let me grab and go without
meeting anyone I know, or who knows me.* It had been a horribly hard day, and my moodiness was elevated due to
many frustrating menopausal moments.

My basket began to fill with toilet paper, Kleenex, and

paper towels as I pushed toward the pet products. Pausing to check the sale price on kitty litter and designer cat food, I got that all-too-familiar feeling. *Okay, stand still. Hold on, ignore that tabletop water feature at the end of the aisle.* As I lifted a twenty-pound bag of kitty litter, the urge instantly became too strong. *I gotta go! I gotta go right now!* Taking a deep breath to get my bearings, and also to avoid an accident, I did a U-turn to the back of the store. *Please God, let there be an open stall,* I prayed. I parked my cart by the stand of old-lady canes and waddled through the door to the women's restroom. God must have been listening, as the restroom was empty.

I took care of my business then returned to my waiting cart. *Now, where was I on my list? Pelligrino, ah, straight ahead on aisle four.* I picked up three bottles and added them to the cart. Pushing onward, I wasn't but halfway up aisle four when that "light-bulb" went off in my brain, AGAIN! I had this sinking feeling that bladder control was becoming a menopausal issue, which was apropos, considering I was surrounded by disposable diapers, feminine hygiene products, incontinence supplies, and bottled water.

Feeling as though my security depended upon my poise (sorry for the play on words), I knew it was time to check out the "grandma" diapers. I looked both ways first to confirm I was alone, then pretended to look at the Pampers, which were next to the incontinence products.

I became confused studying all the products and had a hard time deciding which one to try. *Which is better? Super absorbent, ultra long, light pads? Or adult pull-ups that fit and feel like underwear? Or adjustable ones with and without buttons? How about worry-free with odor control? And what about the all-important disposable? Do I need super, long, or special blue lining? What's with this product that can be used by both men and women? I always thought pink was for girls and blue, for boys.* God knows there was no way I was going to ask the grocery staff for help selecting the right diaper!

I almost settled on getting the Poise pads, but they didn't have wings, which I preferred. Exasperated with not knowing what to purchase—and more so due to the fact that I *had* to purchase these things in the first place—I decided to return later that night just before closing. *Good plan! I can get the forty pounds of kitty litter, then bury the Poise pads beneath it!*

I exited aisle four and headed for the deli. Too late to cook dinner, I picked up a rotisserie chicken and some potato salad, then headed for checkout. I did return later to finish all my shopping—and I mean *all* of it.

Each night, I pray that my menopausal body and soul settles into a more serene routine, one without valleys, hills, or even those constant waterfalls.

Nancy Withers

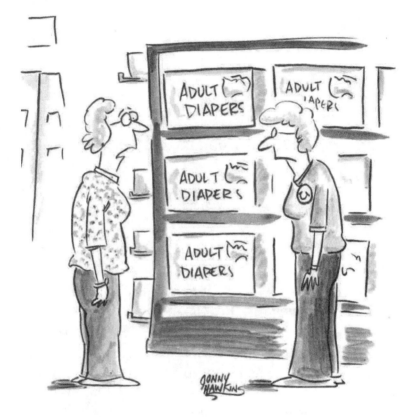

"Do you have any with invisible panty lines?"

A Case of Mistaken Identity

*To make mistakes is human; to stumble is com-
monplace; to be able to laugh at yourself is
maturity.*

William Arthur Ward

Jeannie and I had shared a delightful dinner before
heading to our Bible study. We talked about our families,
laughed about being in the menopausal years of forgetfulness, confusion, and bifocals. And we discussed the "hereafter." You know, when you go into another room and
then try to remember what you went there for in the first
place. But, aside from a few wrinkles, gray hairs, and minor
aches, we were just thankful to be alive and happy.

By the time we left the restaurant and walked across the
parking lot that Tuesday evening in October, it had grown
dark and quite cool. I opened the car door and settled in
the passenger side of the front seat. Pulling my jacket
tighter to ward off the chill, I buckled the seatbelt and
began to take notice of my surroundings. *Gee,* I thought to
myself, *I didn't notice this beautiful wood-grain design before.*
Rubbing my fingers along the dashboard, I thought,

Jeannie must have cleaned and waxed the interior last weekend. Looking down at the console, I noticed a beautiful pair of brown leather gloves. They were so soft and luxurious that I couldn't resist the urge to try them on and see how they looked. After admiring the gloves on my hands, it dawned on me that it was taking Jeannie an awfully long time to get in the car.

As I glanced out the driver's side window, I noticed her three cars away with a look of complete and absolute shock on her face. And then she began to laugh hysterically. It took my befuddled mind but a few moments to realize that I was sitting in the wrong car!

I yanked off the gloves, frantically unbuckled the seatbelt, and stumbled out of the car, desperately hoping that the owners were not having dinner in front of the restaurant's large window. By this time, Jeannie, in total amazement that I could have mistaken a BMW for her green Honda, was laughing uncontrollably, tears streaming down her face.

Before the owners of the BMW could materialize, I jumped into Jeannie's car and yelled, "Let's get out of here!" One look at her face, and I, too, convulsed with laughter. We arrived at Bible study, laughing like children, with mascara running down our faces. It took her all of three minutes before she blurted out the story to everyone.

At the end of class, my closing prayer to myself was *Dear God, please help me with my menopause . . . and don't let that BMW be a stolen vehicle, because my fingerprints are all over it!*

Terri Reinhardt

Today's Forecast: Very Dense

A friend is one who knows you and loves you just the same.

Elbert Hubbard

It was a foggy Sunday morning. My friend Helen and I sat in the church educational building counting the Sunday morning offering. After we totaled the amount and completed the deposit slip, we sat back for a moment and engaged in girl talk while sipping coffee.

"Foggy?" Helen questioned as she stared at me over her rather large red, yellow, and blue reading glasses. The look in her eye conveyed both understanding and empathy, the kind of understanding only a woman of her fifty-plus years would be able to give.

"Yes, foggy," I responded with conviction.

As Helen continued to study my face, Thomas and Howard—two men from our church—walked by our table. After hearing only this part of our conversation, they stopped briefly to speak to us.

Thomas lifted a hot cup of coffee to his lips and said, "Yes, it sure is foggy today. It was so foggy this morning I could hardly see the road ahead of me on my way to church." With this said, Thomas and Howard made their way to the table across the building where others sat waiting to start the adult Sunday School class.

Helen and I silently smiled at one another until they were out of earshot. Then we started giggling. These two men, in all of their male experience, could not possibly know we were not referring to the weather conditions outside. We were discussing my recent cognitive condition; I had been describing to Helen how my thinking had become so confused and unfocused, that it was more than cloudy, it was "foggy."

I had read that "foggy thinking" was a normal symptom of menopause. It just doesn't seem fair. As if hot flashes, night sweats, and mood swings weren't enough of an initiation into the "Mature Woman Club," now I had to also have lapses of memory and unclear thinking!

It seemed to have occurred suddenly. One day I was a fairly sharp and alert person, and the next day I couldn't even remember the names of people I had known for a lifetime. This forgetfulness is very embarrassing, but I have been told by my post-menopausal women friends that it's just a phase and will pass. My poor husband certainly is ready for this phase to be over. He has had to come to my rescue three times over the last two months after I somehow locked my keys in the car.

When Sunday school was over, many of us left the building together, locking the door behind us. As we bid each other a good day and a wish for a great week ahead, Howard said to Thomas, "I sure hope this fog lifts soon."

"Me, too!" I emphatically whispered to Helen, while giving her a hug.

And again, we giggled like two schoolgirls.

Jane Wiatrek

Keep Looking Up

I received a free magazine-ette in the mail the other day. It's one of those little half-sized publications. It came in a protective plastic wrap, as though the contents were precious enough to warrant that extra dose of precaution. The cover hinted at all sorts of health-related topics inside, and since, for some inexplicable reason, I've become fascinated with discussions about estrogen and blood pressure and the evils of salt, I decided to sit right down and peruse my new gift. But when I opened the cover, I saw that about every other page was a tear-out advertisement for something or another.

Since I had an opening in my schedule at that exact moment, I took to pulling out those advertisements. I was a little curious to see exactly how small the magazine-ette would become once it was pared down to actual content. Midway through my purging, I came upon an advertisement for Doubleday's Large Print Book Club. Large Print. I did a double-take, and then I thought, *Why would someone send me a magazine with an offer for a book club that catered to those needing large print?* It then occurred to me that everything I'd read to that point had been in a comfortable, large print. The table of contents, ads, articles—all had been printed larger than your normal publication. *There has to be a mistake. I'm not old enough for these kinds of offers.* Yes, it's true that I've gained a brown spot or two on my hands, and my knees have begun to sing songs, and at least one night a week I wake to the sensation of "a river runs through it." But aside from those oddities, I'm still young. *Surely,* I thought, *this thing got placed in the wrong mailbox.* I found the one-page "You're invited" sheet that had been stuck inside the protective plastic cover and looked at the address label on the bottom, but even with my arms stuck way out, I couldn't get the label far enough away to read. Grabbing my reading glasses, I checked again. My name was typed right there in minuscule letters.

I'd been targeted, identified, zeroed-in on. What did this mean? Did it mean that any day now, the girl down at Golden Corral would stop asking if anyone in our party got the senior discount and just give it to me instead?

I wondered if all the forty-four-year-olds on my street got the magazine. Or maybe one of my sisters turned me in. They seem to delight in teasing me about the length of my arms and the lessening of my vision.

Yes, all right, I'll admit it. Stop badgering. I'm farsighted. I just don't have the ability any more to focus on objects at the drop of a hat. My children will thrust a note under my nose and expect that I can just see it, just like that, just because it's there. Instead, I have to ricochet my head back at lightning speed and put a little distance between me and the must-read material. I have reading glasses tucked in my knitting basket, my basket of books, and the basket of magazines in the bathroom. They're on my nightstand. They're in my office drawer. They're in my purse. More often than not, I have a pair straddling the top edge of my shirt.

But faraway objects, now that's where I excel. I'm not as skilled as my husband, but that's another story. Dave can read the "Made in Taiwan" label on the bottom of a stranger's coffee cup from across a baseball stadium. His vision is disgustingly perfect. But my faraway vision isn't bad. I can sit and look at clouds and mountains all day long, without even breaking a sweat.

He and I were talking over this whole vision issue a few days ago while driving downtown. I happened to be looking at the clouds at that moment.

"I'll tell you what," I said to Dave as I gazed out the window up to the heavens, "I'll take farsightedness over nearsightedness any day. I don't know what I'd do if I couldn't see the sky."

Over the last few years, I've learned I can't get enough of that sight. There's just something about gazing upward that calms me. Whatever comparatively unworthy thing I'm currently fretting over becomes automatically minimized by the sight of all that billowy beauty drifting overhead.

I see a spiritual lesson in that—and no, "see" was not intended as a pun. If I had to choose, I'd rather have a clear focus on heaven than on the here-and-now. I'd rather set my eyes on eternity than on the temporal. It's so easy to get spiritually nearsighted and focus our eyes solely on the things we can touch and taste and feel, even those unpleasant experiences like night sweats and creaky knees, while completely forgetting there's a sky beyond this earth and a heaven waiting to welcome us.

The truth is, growing older is much less painful when you keep *forever* in your sights.

Shannon Woodward

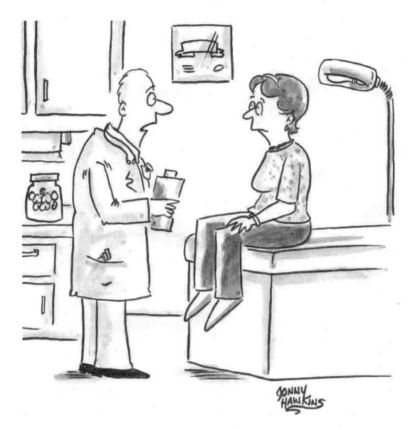

"The good news, Mrs. Dehlman,
is that your hindsight is still 20/20."

Lost in the CD Aisles

If at first you don't succeed, you're running about average.

M. H. Alderson

With so many other decisions that were happening during my mood swings, hot flashes, and crying spells, finding a new vehicle seemed like a good change. That was, until I got to the lot with my husband. It wasn't hard to find something that we liked, but leaving the old family van with all the memories became a bit of a problem for me. I cried all the way home from the dealership.

Although high in miles, the van was in good condition. But we were back to two people; the kids were on their own, and we didn't need a large vehicle. Leaving that old van in the lot caused some unexpected feelings. I wasn't just "leaving" the van, I was saying goodbye to special memories—all the years driving to and from baseball games and band practices and then moving our oldest daughter to her college dorm. This new, smaller minivan we just purchased wasn't part of the family, and it didn't even have a place for a cassette player! Now I would have to figure out this CD player! I really don't like change at all.

I waited to purchase a CD until the very last thing on my list that day. I would have preferred the cassette. I remember making the change from records to cassettes, and it took me a while to get used to that!

"Get with it, Mom," our son admonished over the telephone. "They have oldies on CDs now. Times are changing. You'll love that new player!" he laughed. It wasn't funny. My other cars had radios, and the last two had cassette players.

For that reason it made me wonder what I was doing in the CD aisles. I walked up to a salesclerk and asked, "Do you have anything by Johnny Mathis?"

"Is he country music or pop?" she asked.

"He isn't either." I couldn't believe it. They didn't know Johnny! "He sang 'Small World' and 'Chances Are.'" I waited for a reaction.

"Nope, never heard of him." She looked like she felt sorry for me.

"Okay, I'll just look around a bit. Are these CDs the right size for a car player?" I asked.

"They are unless you have something we aren't aware of. And they'll work on your player at home too," she smiled.

I looked for a name that I knew. There was nothing by Pat Boone or Ricky Nelson. What was this? I went to the aisle that said "pop tunes" and I was lost again! I saw a CD by Natalie Cole and asked another salesclerk, "Do you have anything by her dad, Nat King Cole?"

"Well, we can look his name up in the music archives," she replied.

"Okay, I'm going to keep looking. Will you let me know if you find the old guy in your archives?" I wasn't doing research for a hero from the Revolutionary War. Nat had died young, but I remembered his music.

I thought of all my records at home. My 45 rpm records never cost more than a dollar, and the LPs, depending on the year, were more. But these had $16.95 written on them, and I had never heard of the singers.

I thought I'd pick up the tempo a bit and try to find something by The Fifth Dimension, Burt Bacharach, or Dean Martin. I asked the young man next to me. "Do you know where the Dean Martin CDs are?"

"Is he that Italian dude? I think they have a section for *foreign*," he said and walked away. I stared at the back of his head. Dean didn't sing in Italian, he sang in English. Don't these kids know the greats? I felt a panic attack coming on, and heat was starting to take residence in my face and neck!

My gal came back. "No, we don't have anything by Nat King Cole, just Natalie Cole. Is there something else you'd like to find?"

I thought about asking if she had any Motown classics, but decided she might think I was referring to a new type of car.

"I think I'm all set," I told the sales girl. I picked up a CD by Barry Manilow and tossed it into my cart.

When I got home, my hubby wondered how the shopping had gone.

"I felt like I was having a panic attack in the CD aisle," I replied. "Do you think I'm asking too much to find an artist I know?"

"Dear, exactly how far back did your song search go?" He knew my love for the oldies. I didn't comment further. One has priorities in life. I grew up during the '50s and '60s and belonged to a number of fan clubs. I was loyal.

The next evening, when my husband came home, he had a package for me. I eagerly opened my gift from the sweetest guy in the world and was overjoyed to see a number of CDs by some of my favorite singers. "Where did you find these?" I asked. "At a store near my office," he said. "And now we're going out to the minivan to learn how to work the CD player." He grabbed a CD and my hand and led the way. After we went over how to load the CD player, I told him I'd try it out, and he happily gave me the keys and stood aside. I was driving my new vehicle around the area when a song from my past came on the CD; it was, "Baby, You've Got What It Takes," a duet by a couple of great singers. I opened all the windows and turned up the volume. I felt young again. I knew a hot flash might appear within moments, but right then I was allowing the breeze to kiss my cheeks. My soul felt happy. Perhaps that is the way it should be, to enjoy the moments of life and to cherish each one, however it comes.

Diane Dean White

Oh Lord

I don't mind the hot flashes
Or the sweat that pours and drips.
The ceiling fan is on all night
And there's chocolate on my lips.

I don't mind the elbow brace,
Or the joints so stiff and sore.
The ibuprofen makes me smile
At games I even score.

I don't mind the aching back
Or the mood swings off the wall.
I don't even mind the simple fact
That I used to be quite tall.

I don't mind the eyeglasses,
The dental crowns fit me fine.
There's just one little thing I miss,
Oh Lord, I miss my mind.

Patricia Lorenz

READER/CUSTOMER CARE SURVEY

CG5G

We care about your opinions! Please take a moment to fill out our online Reader Survey at **http://survey.hcibooks.com.**
As a **"THANK YOU"** you will receive a **VALUABLE INSTANT COUPON** towards future book purchases as well as a **SPECIAL GIFT** available only online! Or, you may mail this card back to us and we will send you a copy of our exciting catalog with your valuable coupon inside.

First Name	MI.		Last Name
Address			
State	Zip	City	Email

1. Gender
❑ Female   ❑ Male

2. Age
❑ 8 or younger
❑ 9-12   ❑ 13-16
❑ 17-20   ❑ 21-30
❑ 31+

3. Did you receive this book as a gift?
❑ Yes   ❑ No

4. Annual Household Income
❑ under $25,000
❑ $25,000 - $34,999
❑ $35,000 - $49,999
❑ $50,000 - $74,999
❑ over $75,000

5. What are the ages of the children living in your house?
❑ 0 - 14   ❑ 15+

6. Marital Status
❑ Single   ❑ Married
❑ Divorced   ❑ Widowed

7. How did you find out about the book?
(please choose one)
❑ Recommendation
❑ Store Display
❑ Online
❑ Catalog/Mailing
❑ Interview/Review

8. Where do you usually buy books?
(please choose one)
❑ Bookstore
❑ Online
❑ Book Club/Mail Order
❑ Price Club (Sam's Club, Costco's, etc.)
❑ Retail Store (Target, Wal-Mart, etc.)

9. What subject do you enjoy reading about the most?
(please choose one)
❑ Parenting/Family
❑ Relationships
❑ Recovery/Addictions
❑ Health/Nutrition
❑ Christianity
❑ Spirituality/Inspiration
❑ Business Self-help
❑ Women's Issues
❑ Sports

10. What attracts you most to a book?
(please choose one)
❑ Title
❑ Cover Design
❑ Author
❑ Content

TAPE IN MIDDLE; DO NOT STAPLE

BUSINESS REPLY MAIL

FIRST-CLASS MAIL   PERMIT NO 45   DEERFIELD BEACH, FL

POSTAGE WILL BE PAID BY ADDRESSEE

Chicken Soup for the Soul in Menopause
3201 SW 15th Street
Deerfield Beach, FL 33442-9875

FOLD HERE

Comments

Do you have your own Chicken Soup story
that you would like to send us?
Please submit at: **www.chickensoup.com**

3

IT'S TIME

*God grant me the serenity to accept
the things I cannot change,
the courage to change the things I can,
and the wisdom to know the difference.*

Reinhold Niebuhr

No More Babies

*I may not have gone where I intended to go, but
I think I have ended up where I intended to be.*

Douglas Adams

I can remember the exact moment—where I was, what
I was wearing, even how my hair was styled—when I
truly realized that I was a menopausal woman.

It was in the cereal aisle of a busy supermarket, and I
was passing a young mother with one of those babies
straight out of a catalog: thatch of blonde hair, enormous
blue eyes, dimpled arms, sturdy little legs. I stared at that
mother and baby for a long moment, then felt tears spring
to my eyes. *No more babies. Not for me. Not ever again,* I said
to myself. I left my cart in the aisle and bolted outside to
my car, where I sat and wept.

I was forty-four years old, had three children, a wonderful life, an interesting career as a journalist—and a
body that would never again carry a child. And suddenly,
I felt the total impact of that reality. I was blindsided. Mind
you, I hadn't planned to have any more babies. Oh sure, it
would have been nice to finally get that little boy my

husband and I would have called "Jonathan" after greeting
Jill, then Amy, then Nancy; it was after Nancy's birth we
realized that a gender trend was definitely developing.
But back in that era—the early 1980s—women in their
forties weren't in the full bloom of pregnancies the way
they are now. And presumably enlightened doctors might
even have counseled against so "risky" a proposition. But
emotions don't go to college. And what pushed forth that
day in the supermarket was some deep, almost paralyz-
ing, sense of loss.

I loved having babies. I even loved being pregnant. And
slipping into menopause rather early and quite suddenly
had felt vaguely like an ambush. How ironic that I was the
last girl in my crowd to get "it," as we euphemistically
called menstruation, and the first to go through "the
change," another term my generation inherited. In both
instances, it felt odd.

For months, I never told my husband about my meltdown in the supermarket. But I thought about it often and
briefly found myself avoiding places where babies would
logically be. Inevitably, of course, they seemed to be
everywhere. For months, I had dreams of tiny ones. I
didn't need Dr. Freud to tell me that my subconscious was
working through something vast and deep.

And then, just as unexpectedly as it had begun, my sadness lifted. Life was back on an even keel, and I could
rejoice once again at the sight of babies. I could reach out
and touch their fat cheeks and delicious little arms and
feel pleasure.

Yes, I was a menopausal woman. There would be no
more babies for me. And at last, that was exactly where I
belonged. My soul had come into alignment with my
body.

It didn't hurt that within the next few years, I would
receive the spectacular gift of motherhood-once-removed,

that euphoric, love-crazed state called grandparenthood. It didn't hurt that we even got some boys in the mix— none named Jonathan, alas, but oh what treasures!

And just recently, I stopped in my tracks at the super- market to admire another of those dream babies. It was in the cereal aisle again. This time, I felt nothing but soaring joy at the sight of this perfect little specimen in her snug- gly, close to her mother's heart. That mother and I, perfect strangers, smiled at one another as we shared that sister- hood we mothers automatically have. Without words, we somehow spoke volumes about what it is to bear and love a child.

And menopause can't change that one bit.

Sally Friedman

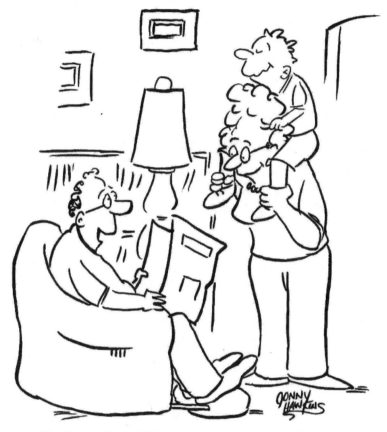

"And you thought menopause meant the end of child-bearing, eh Grandma?"

Accepting the Inevitable

I'm hot; then I'm not,
and the heat rushes through.
The flashes pass by,
and I'm left feeling blue.

They say life gets better.
They tell me to wait.
I want to believe them;
resigned to my fate.

A bladder too small,
and hips growing bigger;
the water retained
could fill the Nile River.

My skin is so dry.
And I'm losing my hair.
I frequently feel
like I'm not quite all there.

Moody and restless,
forgetful and late;

night sweats are common,
and I keep gaining weight.

I'm sleeping too little.
I'm sleeping too much.
Life is changing too fast,
but not fast enough.

Hormones are bad.
No, hormones are good.
Take what you can.
No, take what you should:

Enzymes and calcium,
vitamins B, C, and E.
What I really need now
is a nutrition degree.

Black cohosh and ginseng,
primrose and dong quai;
I've learned a new language.
There's one reason why.

I'm too young to suffer.
What could be the cause?
It's my new pal Peri:
Perimenopause!

Ava Pennington

Scary Numbers

I was one of the lucky ones who had never been traumatized by a birthday. That couldn't last forever, of course, and when the birthday blues finally struck they felt more like the birthday black-and-blues!

How did I escape for so long? I wondered to myself. When the big 3-0 rolled around, I was getting married. I was focused on the future rather than the feelings of fading youth. My life was still carefree, and I didn't look any different than I had in my twenties. Thirty was just an abstract number that didn't apply to me.

When forty loomed on the horizon, I was giving birth. Babies are not only fun to have around, but they make great fashion accessories for moms over forty. Amidst the camouflage of a drooling infant, people tend to lump you into the category of "young mother." It's easy to be in denial about your age when you are just embarking on a decade of Disney and dolls. In such a jolly setting, the big 4-0 didn't scare me in the least. In fact, not only was I not trying to hide the numbers, I didn't even mind volunteering the information.

But that kind of naïve optimism couldn't last forever. The fabulous forties were flying by, and I was blissfully oblivious to the numbers piling up behind me. I was oblivious, that is, until the number forty-nine rolled around.

Suddenly, it was as if a car was racing toward me at 100 miles an hour. I wanted to slam on the brakes. But there are no brakes in the vehicle of life, only a limited warranty. I was moving forward at top speed whether I liked it or not and heading for a crash. Soon, I would have sagging bumpers and flat tires. I would be a wreck.

For the very first time I felt empathy for all those afflicted with the thirty-something and forty-something blues. The prospect of turning fifty was really getting me down. For this reason, I made the most of forty-nine, clinging to the number "four" like it was a lifeboat. As the days sped by, I began to panic. Physical changes were starting to creep in, but I refused to acknowledge the "M" word, secretly referring to it as "many paws," a joke I shared with my aging Chihuahua. For me, the physical symptoms seemed like small potatoes compared with the psychological impact of kissing my youth goodbye.

My anxieties were aggravated by the media. If fifty was supposed to be the new thirty, why did the media treat it like the new eighty! From life insurance to health-care, all the commercials seemed to begin with the same outlandish phrase, "If you're between the ages of fifty and eighty, this message is for you. . . . "

Could fifty and eighty actually be part of the same demographic? When you're still buying your jeans at the Gap and doing cartwheels in the backyard with your grade-schoolers, retirement plans and health-care products seem like futuristic curiosities. It is hard to retain such youthful optimism when advertisers keep bombarding you with the need to plan your own funeral.

Even leisure activities offered no refuge. While watching the movie *Sunset Boulevard,* I was confronted with the image of archetypal decay—Norma Desmond, the faded movie star—a woman of fifty! I ran to the mirror and studied my reflection; was I ready for the waxworks? In a panic, I planned to buy stock in Oil of Olay. If need be, I would submerge myself in a vat of the moisturizer!

Despite it all, I tried to keep my spirits up and ignore the negative hype. D-Day arrived, and I vowed I wasn't going to get psyched out by a number. Then it happened. It came in the mail on my birthday, and it wasn't a coupon for a free scoop of ice cream. It was a subscription to AARP, a magazine from and for the American Association of Retired Persons! I snapped. It's hard to keep your chin up when it's starting to double! I faced the day like a zombie. I felt like I was walking the plank.

Though birthday plans were in place, I was numb. As we drove off to a nearby ski resort, I was sleepwalking through the day. I just couldn't shake the unsettling feelings. The big number had been haunting me for months, and now it had arrived. *Was this really the end of my youth?*

Then, the strangest thing happened. After we arrived at the lodge and my daughter and I took off in the snow, everything changed in an instant. It was her first time on skis. She was having the time of her life. I was having the time of my life, and my husband and youngest daughter were cheering us on from a chalet balcony. I forgot about numbers altogether. We stayed on the slopes for hours. The feelings of gloom and doom had vanished into the crisp, snowy air. Not only did I enjoy the day, I got through it without breaking my hip! It occurred to me that joy strikes like lightning and isn't tied to age. If I was having the time of my life, it didn't matter what time it was—chronologically speaking.

Older isn't necessarily better than younger, but it isn't always worse. In fact, on certain occasions it can actually be better. If the clock had stopped at forty-nine, I would have missed the fun I had on the scariest birthday of my life.

So from now on, I will leave the numbers to the mathematicians and go back to being my old self again. My younger old self, that is.

E. Mitchell

The Pinup Girl

My husband reminded me to go grocery shopping. I hate shopping for food and agree to it only because it's my job and obligation as a good wife, although I never read it in the marriage vows. *Do you promise to love, honor, and do the food shopping?* But every week since I've started school at Florida International University, a late-in-life decision I admit, the conversation goes like this:

"Honey, don't you think it's time to get plastic bags, ice cream—the chunky kind—and dog food? Oh yeah, bread, ham, cheese, and steaks. . . . "

Well, you get the idea.

On Friday of last week I found myself at Publix sprinting down the dairy aisle. I felt a cart close behind me, but I didn't stop to turn around. My focus was to get in and out as quickly as possible. I have been known to throw a container discus-style from fifty feet into my food cart—call me Michael Jordan. (Hint: Cold cuts fly especially well, and they don't splatter when they hit. Or you miss.)

I moved on to the meat section and felt the rush of adrenaline; I was almost done. Reaching for the rib eye steaks, I heard an older female's voice, "You should be a model. Someone should take a picture and send it in to one of those magazines. I mean, everything about you—your hair, your face, your body, they all work."

Well, what could I do? If someone tells you that you look like a model, especially if you're over fifty, you stop to talk with them. I wanted to kiss her, actually. I didn't think I'd looked that great when I left the house that morning. Now she was telling me I looked glamorous. She was about seventy years old, and she looked darn good herself. Her hair was gray but well-styled, and she had a petite body and well-shaped jaw line with high cheek bones.

I tried to sound modest. I'm not sure if it worked. What I really wanted to tell her was that I'd been a model most of my life. Not anything big-time, like Cindy Crawford, but in my thirties I'd had enough small jobs to earn a living. I was the ditzy brunette who said, "You'll love it at Levitz." But now I was older. In the last few years the economy dropped; when that happens, so do advertising campaigns. The terrorist attack on 9/11 didn't help. At fifty, I'm in a nonexistent category: too old to play the slice-of-life housewife and too young to sell pharmaceuticals. My next big earning market will be in my sixties, if I survive and am still breathing. Instead of crying in my beer, I decided to stop waiting for agents to call with job offers and registered for college courses, including creative writing. *But what did this woman care about my modeling career?*

She stared at my face, not willing to let the subject go. "No, really. You look good."

"You mean for my age," I said. I knew that's what she really meant.

"How old are you?" she asked.

"Fifty-three."

"I never would have known if you didn't tell me."

"We both look great for our ages."

I guess that was the wrong thing to say. She smiled

searching for the right words—her lips formed a round hole—but nothing came out. Then I realized that I'd made her uncomfortable; I tried to look at the steaks in the freezer, anywhere but her face. She leaned over her cart. "I've been out in the sun much of my life. All of this," she pointed to her face with her index finger, "is wrinkled now."

I saw her eyes travel back to another world, and I waited patiently for her story. She didn't disappoint me.

"I worked for my father. We used to raise chickens. I'd go out and collect the eggs while the hens were sitting. One day someone took a picture of me in a big straw hat and sent it in to a magazine. It appeared overseas."

I don't know why, but I could suddenly see how she must have looked back then. Long brown hair flowing in the summer breeze, teeth glistening in the sunshine, and Betty Grable-shorts that showed all of her curves. She was beautiful.

"One of my friends called and asked, 'Aida, what are you doing overseas?' I laughed and told them the picture was taken here in Miami. I'd never left. I'd never been outside of Florida. But there I was, overseas in a magazine. Them boys were pinning that picture up of me over their beds at night. Can you imagine that? I was a pinup girl."

I felt a lump form in my throat. I was witnessing a great moment in time. She was talking about World War II. She had been the reason why so many of our boys, now our grandfathers, had come back home. She was their inspiration.

There are days when you have to do things you don't want to do. If you do them, sometimes there is a reward at the end—if you take the time to see it. She was mine.

Joyce Newman Scott

Living in the Hot Lane

I feel it approaching, the way you know when a train is about to pull into the station before you see it. Two seconds later it comes roaring in, the ol' hot flash express, filling me with its suddenness, its engine steaming inside me. I hope it will pass through quickly, and I'll be able to get on with what I am doing. If not, I will have to carry on anyway. Life doesn't stop just because I'm living in the hot lane.

I have tried to describe to my husband what a hot flash feels like, but there is really no way he can know without experiencing it. What he does feel is the outer manifestation. He says I am "swampy." And he is right. Rivulets of sweat flow down my body, pooling in any small indentation: the crook of an elbow, back of my knees, between my breasts.

I am grateful that I work at home. I can get up from my computer and jump into the tub when it gets too uncomfortable. I don't have to worry about leaving a puddle on my chair at an important client meeting. I have been known to stick my head inside the freezer when it really gets to me.

One friend, who does go to client meetings, never lets

on when she is burning up. She has, however, allowed her hair to grow a little longer so she can cover her ears. They turn bright pink when she flashes.

Another friend is also experiencing this transition. Her husband says she turns the air conditioner thermostat so low at night that icicles form in his nostrils. I have no sympathy. He knows where to find the extra blankets.

The standard advice for flashers is to take hormone replacement therapy. But it is not for everyone. Not for my friend with a heart condition, or for the one with a family history of ovarian cancer. Not for me with my alternative philosophy.

So we balance wild yam and isoflavones, primrose oil and dong quai, looking for the combinations that work for us. And we talk to each other, sharing our stories and laughing. A lot. One thing we discovered is that none of us feel our femininity is threatened by the knowledge that one day soon we will not be able to have children. We don't feel any less desirable. Our sex drive is still in gear. It just isn't an issue.

And we don't see this as a disease that needs to be cured. It is just a natural part of the maturing process. Some of us feel it more acutely than others but we are individuals and bound to vary in our responses to this time of life. We don't deny what we are going through; we work through it with information and accommodation and intelligence.

What we have noticed is that our sisterhood has deepened. We cannot talk about such intimate things without drawing closer. And that has many benefits. We see how we have grown over the years because we are no longer afraid or embarrassed to tell the truth. With truth comes power. We know who we are now. We accept ourselves with all the flaws and inconsistencies that come with living actively.

So what if living in the hot lane has its inconveniences? They will pass eventually, but the joy we women have in each other will remain. We are getting the better part of the deal.

Ferida Wolff

Enlightenment of a
Spandex-Clad Eavesdropper

Every exit is an entry somewhere.

Tom Stoppard

The experience was always so excruciating and fraught with potential psychic assault that I had postponed it as long as possible. It was only because my trip to Hawaii was swiftly approaching, thus necessitating the purchase, that I even considered the agonizing activity. Yes, for sheer emotional drama, trying on swimsuits was up there with root canals, incarceration, and various forms of public humiliation.

In truth, a swimwear purchase was no joyride even in my younger years. Now, however, menopause had left its all too evident markers upon my body. Facing myself, scantily clothed, in a fluorescent-lit dressing room replete with full-length mirrors was almost more than I could bear without heavy sedation.

Nonetheless, I am an optimist and I was determined to find a suit that would flatter my expanded figure. So, after repeating several uplifting affirmations of love and acceptance of myself in all of my matronly magnificence, I headed off to the store. Locating the swimsuit department, I swiftly strolled past the size-two bikinis and headed for the mature woman's section—the one featuring dark colors, industrial-strength spandex, and swimskirts cleverly designed for concealment.

After making my selections, I entered that chamber of horrors, aka the dressing room, to face my fate. Astonishingly, I was in for a rather pleasant surprise. Technology does have its good side for once, as I was able to squeeze my ample hips into the swimsuit. The result wasn't all that bad. It was evident that major improvements to the muscle-power inherent within elastic and its subsequent clones had evolved over the years. In fact, the suit compacted my flesh with a brawny force so strong that I was pressed and squeezed within an inch of my life. I did realize that I would be unable to draw a full breath, so I couldn't save myself should I be drowning, but, all in all, I was happy. I even decided to venture out of my curtain-draped cubicle to brave the real test—the "cheek check" in the three-way mirror down the hall.

It was then that I heard them. I parted the curtains just enough to spot two giggling teenagers, with taut, perfect bodies, carrying in their selected suits. I quickly closed my peephole and swiftly hid myself in the dark recesses of my cubicle, thankful for a place to conceal my barely clothed body. It had only been a matter of seconds, or I would have been caught observing my backside, reflected with tri-angled grandeur in that ghastly mirror, fully exposed to laughing teenage eyes and smirks of disdain.

Shortly after I huddled silently in my draped refuge, however, something remarkable happened. This unexpected encounter became a mind-blowing lesson that totally transformed my outlook on life.

Unaware that I was there, the girls ceased their giggling

and started swapping tales of boyfriends, girlfriends, and some real instances of teenage angst. Their feelings seemed openly raw as they shared stories of social slights, rebuffs, and even betrayals from their so-called friends. More amazingly, as they tried on their suits, they each expressed anxiety and even pain about their bodies.

"I'm a disgusting whale!" whined one.

Her friend moaned in reply, "Like you should talk. I look like a fat pig with no boobs and zits on my back."

I was astounded. These girls, with their unlined skin, firm flesh, and slender bodies, believed their looks to be woefully substandard and "gross," while I viewed them as youthful perfection. They focused only on their imperceptible flaws, and each seemed to suffer major distress and insecurity.

Then it hit me—no way would I ever want to go back there! Mercifully, I now benefited from the buffer of several decades between my present reality and my own teenage years. Remembrance of that time had, thankfully, softened into bits and pieces and the hazy mists of recollections from long ago. The conversation I was now overhearing, however, struck me in my gut as it evoked my own teen feelings of self-consciousness, inadequacy, and major, painful mood swings.

How grateful I became in my eavesdropping-induced reveries to realize that I now enjoyed the wonders of fullfledged menopause! My days passed pleasantly and productively, and I enjoyed my many activities. I no longer experienced hormonal moodiness, nor did I obsess over every perceived slight, omission, or inadvertent social snub. I had ceased my slavish need to please others and even learned to say "no" when it suited me. I was more assertive, more confident, and far more self-possessed than ever before. I realized, with a rush of joy, that I really and truly liked myself!

Even more, I recognized how happy I was with my well-worn, puckered, and full-figured body. This remarkable organism had experienced love, borne a child, remained healthy, and served me well all these years. In fact, I became so enthralled with myself that I decided to venture out of my hiding place and strut down the hallway to that three-way mirror in all my vibrating glory!

So, taking as deep a breath as possible, given the crushing force of the swimsuit, I parted the curtains and marched regally down to the mirror. The girls were just leaving and walked by me with nary a glance. There were no smirks or rolls of the eyes. They were far too engaged in their own conversation to even notice me.

When I later approached the checkout with my selected suit, I recognized that the cashier was a woman about my age. As she removed the plastic sensor, she remarked: "This one is really attractive. With your coloring, I bet it looks great on you."

"Well, thank you," I replied. "I'm really pleased."

And, as I left the store I realized that, in every fiber of my being, I truly was.

Mary Eileen Williams

An Ounce of Dignity

We can let circumstances rule us, or we can take charge and rule our lives from within.

Earl Nightingale

Having gone all through my life with an upbeat, laid-back, go-with-the-flow attitude, I rarely gave a thought to menopause or its effects. Menopause was something that happened to much older ladies, and I had just turned fifty. I could never attribute any grumpiness or anger to PMS, mood swings, or hormones. I just recognized I was having a bad day and things would soon look up. And, except for unusually long labors, both of my pregnancies were pleasant and uneventful. Menopause? No problem.

Because of an ovarian fibroid tumor, I was given injections once a month for three months to stop my production of estrogen. This would reduce the size of the fibroid for a less invasive type of surgery to remove the tumor and perform a subtotal hysterectomy. Thus began my abrupt and swift journey into the "the change of life."

My normally cheerful personality came to a screeching halt. While I admit to the usual emotional or sentimental tears, I soon became a test pilot for waterproof mascara! While driving to work in rush-hour traffic, I would hear a sad song on the country radio station and the waterworks would start. By the time I arrived at work, my eyes were red, swollen, and puffy, and I was emotionally drained for no reason! The more I thought about my crying episodes, the more upset I became, and the whole cycle started again.

Had it only been the crying jags I was experiencing, dealing with my changing personality would have been a bit easier. But let's add the lack of concentration, hot flashes, insomnia, and the dreaded night sweats! Oh, I forgot to mention the forgetfulness aspect of menopause. I once did my bi-weekly grocery shopping and pulled into my driveway, when it suddenly dawned on me that I had driven away without my groceries! Fortunately, my grocery cart was still waiting for me in the loading zone.

How could one person sail through life without so much as a mood swing and suddenly end up on a trapeze in her own real-life circus? Some days I'd walked around like a zombie because, after hours of tossing and turning the night before, I would finally fall asleep, only to awake cold and sweaty. And forget going back to sleep right away; by that time, I'm ready to turn down the heat or crank up the air conditioning or crank up the heat and turn down the air conditioning, whichever my fickle body was demanding at the moment. My husband said our home felt like a meat locker, and he half-expected to bump into a side of beef. Yet I was drenched in perspiration. I'm sure I will eventually get back to my normal self, if I can only remember what that was like! But at least the crying has been reduced to the occasional sad song or Hallmark commercial.

All in all, when I consider menopause and how it affects women in a multitude of ways, I am thankful that my symptoms have been relatively mild. I am especially grateful that I have been able to handle them with a touch of grace, an ounce of dignity, and a truckload of humor.

Terri Reinhardt

A Short Trip to Mentalpause

Born with boundless energy, I run naturally in high gear. Even as a teenager, I thought sleep was a waste of time. But one morning about two years ago I awoke as usual at 6 AM and waited for my daily dose of adrenaline to kick in—and it didn't happen! After dragging myself out from under the covers, I remember looking at my husband and wondering why the heck I married him. As I stared into space, I felt as though I was an alien in my own body. I felt weird!

Everything annoyed me—the weather, my children, the dog—everything. I found myself enjoying solitude much more than I ever did. I was constantly tired. I forgot things and had trouble remembering people's names. After three weeks of this "unfocused" feeling, I was convinced insanity was right around the corner.

Then I began to experience all kinds of aches and pains. My back and my knees felt as if they belonged to a ninety-five-year-old woman. I was gaining weight and my periods had become very irregular. I knew then that a trip to the doctor was in order—surely he could tell me what was going on with my normally youthful body!

After two hours of being poked, prodded, and aggravated,

the doctor entered my room grinning like crazy.

"So help me. If you tell me I'm pregnant, I'll kill you," I said.

"No, just the opposite, Marianne. It's just the opposite."

What was the opposite of pregnancy? Senility? Alzheimer's? What? I thought.

"You're in menopause," he stated as if he were happy about it.

"No way, I'm way too young. Something else must be wrong." I was convinced that I was inches away from a nervous breakdown.

My doctor just laughed. I was in menopause. *Where was that? Somewhere near New Jersey?* I sobbed all the way home.

The next few months were torture, mostly self-inflicted. I had refused any hormone treatment because I knew the Doc was wrong. So, when that first "hot flash" hit, I handled it as well as could be expected—from a mad woman!

"Ahhhhh," I bellowed. "I am literally burning up."

I began fanning myself and submerging my wrists under ice water. After that, I began peeling off layers of clothing. I sat in the den wearing just my bra and panties. It was January 14th. And they only got worse. My husband would call before leaving work to make sure I was dressed; his greatest fear was bringing his boss home and having me greet them at the door wearing nothing but a smile!

The family lived in mortal fear of my mood swings. I cried at Coke commercials and burst into laughter at a funeral. The slightest thing could set me off, and I ate as if someone had a gun to my head. But the worst part was I felt old. I waited for a beard and mustache to appear!

Little "mental" slip-ups happened almost daily like locking the car keys in the car, leaving the water running, or forgetting to turn the iron off. One day I actually went to work wearing two different socks. I finally decided it was time for another visit to my doctor.

He placed me on a low-dose hormone patch. Though I began to feel better, the patches had one drawback—they didn't stick very well. I left them everywhere. After starting out on my hip, they would mysteriously end up on my husband, the dog—we never knew when or where a patch would surface. After my daughter wore one to a Girl Scout meeting, I decided another medication would be a good idea.

I began to read everything I could about this "wonderful time in a woman's life!" I wanted to know if anyone had actually survived this trip into "mentalpause." I had serious doubts I could make it through!

After a few months, I found the secret—wine! The doctor suggested that I have two glasses at night with dinner. Even though the wine relaxed me, the symptoms persisted. Now I had a potbelly and my face was breaking out. I needed help! If I was this bad at forty-eight, what the heck was I going to be like at sixty?

I had to get a grip. I changed my diet, cutting way back on the carbs, and began a faithful walking regimen. After a few medication disasters, we finally found one that worked and wasn't shared with the rest of my household. Some of my symptoms were caused by a very large fibroid tumor. I needed a hysterectomy, and just a few weeks after the surgery I began to feel like myself again. I lost weight and gained a healthy outlook on my future. And, I am happy to report, I have yet to gain a beard or mustache.

There's a time in every woman's life when change is unavoidable. I was fortunate to have a supportive husband with a wonderful sense of humor and a dedicated, professional doctor who listened to me. But most of all, I turned my life around, and it is a time of freedom and new beginnings. Have faith in yourself and what you are capable of—it is "your time." Enjoy it!

Marianne LaValle-Vincent

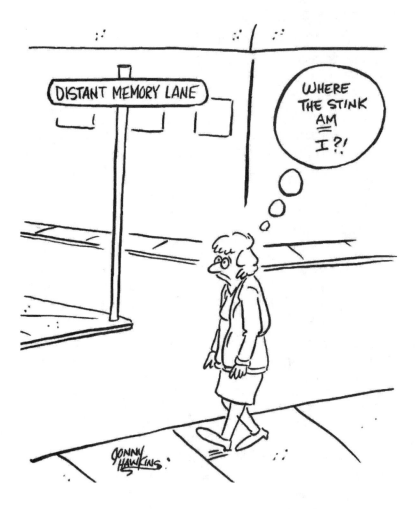

Growing Older

When I look in the mirror what do I see?
Am I just an aging relic of who I used to be?
The hair has grown gray while the hips have
    grown wide,
no trace of the slender figure that gave me much
    pride.

I am now middle aged, stuck in between,
my children are grown yet I still feel eighteen.
Too old to party, for by dusk my energy will fade,
yet I'm too young to surrender to the rocking
    chair brigade.

I've discovered something recently while visiting
    with a friend,
midlife is really an awakening—now that's a mindful
    trend!
When time slows our steps it's old age that we
    blame,
we'd grow old more gracefully by changing the
    rules of the game.

I don't know where I'm going, but I'm sure of where
   I've been,
and, given the chance, I'd do it all over again.
The lines etched across my face will remain forever
   after,
wrinkles born of a life filled with love, joy, and
   laughter.

So, don't let these midlife growing pains be the
   dawn of your demise,
keep in your heart the motto, I am healthy, happy,
   and wise.
And, when you gaze into the mirror that someone
   you will know,
is a seasoned former teenager whose wisdom is
   friend, not foe.

Kathy Whirity

Unsinkable

So this is post-hysterectomy. The little pain I've had, erased by a few doses of Darvocet. I guess it's the avalanche of post-surgical emotions. Not even close to thundering down the slopes of my heart. One of these days, I'll stroll down the feminine hygiene aisle and blissfully pass by tampons and pads while chanting "Free at last, free at last."

And the best news of all: Though the doctor swept my body clean of its uterus, he left two healthy ovaries intact—the lifeboats keeping me from sinking into instant menopause. Does it get any better than this? Now that I've tallied everything right about my life and have comfortably settled into my parents' townhouse to recuperate, I've started to feel like a new woman.

That is, until I see my "sister."

Walking around the basement in my sweats, I see the old Frigidaire refrigerator humming away in the furnace room. The rounded corners, the plump, white body—how familiar she is. My parents purchased her when I was three months old, so I've come to think of her as a sister. The Frigidaire and I share many good memories of the fifties and sixties.

And therein lies the reason for the unexpected dip in mood. I had overlooked my age during my tally of all things right. Seeing the fridge reminds me that we've logged fifty years together—half a century.

Goodbye, new-woman feeling.

Okay, so the anesthetic and two days in the hospital have disconnected me from reality, but somewhere I've lost fifty years. Where's that younger face, that carefree sprint past this fridge and out the door to roller-skate or ride bikes? Where are the sharp eyes, the supple skin? I have bifocals now (thank God for progressive lenses). Skin puckers on my elbows and is slowly gathering under my eyes, and graying eyebrows are met with the precision tug of tweezers.

But that's not the worst. Long before surgery, I added *perimenopause* to my vocabulary—a single word that explained multiple oddities in body and behavior. It was like a seismic mood shift that registered 7.5 on the Richter scale, with aftershocks rumbling in slow traffic, long lines, and wherever else I declared people idiots. Insomnia stabbed me awake at odd hours of the night, and I dragged through the next day. My memory spent less and less time remembering why I'd entered a room. My menstrual cycles, once so predictable, alternated between barely there to an overflowing floodgate. When they entered a collision course with fibroid tumors, a hysterectomy was scheduled to stop the monthly madness.

So here I am with the Frigidaire. The gains in recuperation don't seem as great now as I huddle in two ovarian lifeboats. I can float for only so long before they give out, and then I will go into the inevitable: night sweats and hot flashes and weight gain. I'll fan myself till my arms ache and wear sleeveless blouses on twenty-degree days. I'll throw the covers off the bed during the night, gasping for cool air as I soak the sheets. I'll squeeze into clothes that fit so well now, or wear sweats the rest of my life. And somewhere in all the mayhem, the band will be reverently playing "Nearer My God to Thee."

How lucky this Frigidaire is. She's an appliance, not a human being. Her bodily changes are nicks in the handle, smudges on the enamel, and a freezer door sealed with three-inch frost. But, I must admit, she endures without complaint. She hums along, refusing to be defeated by what she can't control.

That helps me. Menopause, I conclude, is inevitable; sinking isn't. Myriads of women have gone through it, so I can survive. Like a midlife Molly Brown, I'll sit in the lifeboats as long as they'll hold. I'll grab the oars and row into the unknown.

Yes, I'm fifty and heading for "the change," and I should make the most of it. If my sister can do it, so can I.

Sherri Langton

Age Is Just a Number

If I have not seen as far as others, it is because there were giants standing on my shoulders.

Harold Abelson

A few weeks before my fortieth birthday, my husband and I visited a favorite eatery for a late-night snack. For months, my spirits had sagged. Earlier in the week I had confided to a friend my fear of aging. "Age is just a number," she reminded me, "Nothing more."

Easy for her to say, but the number wasn't what bothered me. It was much more multifaceted. The slim figure I had managed to inherit from a long line of skinny ancestors started to turn on me. I learned how tiresome it was to keep the pounds from piling on. Were I not so vain, I would, no doubt, be enormous.

And my arms seemed to be getting shorter. Whenever I tried to read the newspaper I saw nothing but a blur of ink. And my toes, protesting years of being forced into spike heels, sprouted unsightly corns and calluses—as protective gear, I suppose.

And then there was the way society as a whole viewed

aging women. From my observations, when they weren't patronizing or mocking them, they ignored them. This only irritated me more when I observed that the same treatment didn't hold true for aging men. Older women were often labeled "elderly," while men enjoyed words like "distinguished" and "sophisticated."

As I brooded about this aging thing, our waitress approached and placed tall glasses of water in front of us. I couldn't help but notice how old she looked. Her hair was coiled into a smooth gray bun, while deep wrinkles spiraled down her face in every direction. The skin on her arms dangled loosely below her sleeves.

Straightening up, she smiled and said, "Hello, my name is Betty, and I will be your waitress tonight. You folks ready to order?"

We ordered, and Betty took our menus, strolling off with a lively step.

She is probably faking it, I thought. *She probably hates her job and can't stand to look at herself in a mirror. With that many wrinkles and that much flab, how else could she feel?*

In a minute, I heard rambunctious laughter coming from behind the counter. Turning, I saw a smooth gray bun moving up and down, in perfect rhythm with the loudest laugh. Betty and a coworker were trembling.

Curious, I found myself watching Betty's every move. Apparently, some of the counter customers were regulars, because occasionally she called out things like, "You need more coffee over there, Harold?" or "Carolyn, your omelet's coming right up, dear."

Whenever an order appeared in the kitchen window, Betty lost no time in collecting the items onto a large round tray, hoisting it above her right shoulder and crossing the room in an unswerving manner. I was entranced by the way she rushed around tables, carrying steaming dishes and pitchers of cold beverages.

As she cleared dirty dishes from a table across the way, the cashier called to her. "Betty, Tom's here." Quickly drying her hands on her apron, Betty rushed to the front, where a tall man, about my age, stood dangling car keys. They hugged and stood there, making conversation. In a minute, Tom pointed toward the glass doors. Betty's gaze followed, and she waved and blew kisses, evidently, to someone waiting in a car.

Their conversation ended, Tom put an arm around Betty's shoulders, gave her another hug, then walked toward the door. As he turned and gave a final wave, she called out, "I love you, son. Drive careful." He nodded and disappeared into the night.

When Betty brought our check, I looked into her face more deeply than I had before, and I was somewhat surprised by my discoveries. Instead of the aging body and gray hair, I saw a woman who laughed easily, a woman who enjoyed her job, a woman who liked her customers, a woman who loved her son, a woman who, in my opinion, had plenty of reasons to frown, but didn't.

I left the restaurant refreshed. Betty had confirmed, once again, that getting old does not mean we cease to influence others. That was evidenced by the smile I wore on my face, as I settled into the car for the drive home.

Dayle Allen Shockley

4

YOU'RE NOT ALONE

Come to the edge
He said. They said: We are afraid.
Come to the edge
He said. They came.
He pushed them, and
they flew.

Guillaume Apollinaire

A Slice of Life

I stepped over Grandpa's old hunting dog, Jake, as he flopped across the back porch, and his only response was the thump-thump-thumping of his tail on the wood planks. The screen door squeaked open and slammed behind me as I tried to focus my eyes to the light in the kitchen. Granny was sliding a pan of cornbread onto a plate, and the old skillet hissed as she eased it into the sudsy sink. Turning, she gave me the heartfelt country welcome I had come to depend on throughout my forty-eight years.

"C'mon in here, honey. I'm so glad you stopped by!"

I hugged Granny and eased into one of the old green vinyl chairs at the table.

"How are you feeling today, Granny?"

"Oh, I reckon I can't complain."

She never did. Granny stood at the sink, a faded apron draped over her ample belly and tied in a neat bow at the back of her calico housedress. Her soft white hair was pulled back into a tight bun, and after eighty-nine years, it had grown thin enough to show hints of her pink scalp underneath. As she leaned, I caught a glimpse of the elastic garters holding up the nylon hose she wore every day.

Every time I came to Granny's kitchen, it felt like coming home. Nothing had changed in it during my growing-up years except for having to replace the refrigerator a few years back. Her trusty cook stove had been rewired but was still "doing its job" as Granny put it. The old green teapot clock still hummed happily on the wall over the stove. The white enamel countertops with the red edging had been chipped a little but were still clean and shiny. And the wallpaper flowers had paled, but overall, it was comforting the same. Just like Granny.

Lately I had been feeling so down, and it was hard to explain why, even to myself. I knew part of it was facing fifty and the big changes in my life—my very empty nest now that all of the kids had left home, my husband's plans for our retirement growing closer and closer, and the way my body and mind seemed to be out to get me.

Granny knew I had these things on my mind, and she had let me talk about them many times over the last few months, giving a sympathetic ear because she knew I didn't talk about myself to many other people but her. As usual for Granny, though, she had not yet given much advice.

"Granny, did you have hot flashes when you were my age?"

"Humph," she grunted, "If'n I did, I never knowed it."

"Did you have night sweats?"

"Yeah, on hot nights, we all sweat!" she laughed.

Today, she sat down beside me at the table, handed me a paring knife and plunked down a big wooden bowl filled with ripe green Granny Smith apples. Granny's steel blue eyes looked knowingly into mine, and she said in her matter-of-fact way, "Hon, I think we need to make us an apple pie. You peel 'em while I make the crust."

I began to turn the fruit in my hand, the knife unwinding the long curls of apple peel. She walked over and began gathering the things around her kitchen she needed, cradling them in her apron by holding up the bottom corners in one hand. She methodically arranged them on the chipped tabletop and began to mix the crust, but her eyes were on me. "What's in your heart, child?"

As I peeled and cored and sliced the apples, I began to tell her again how I hated the thought of the "change of life" when it didn't seem like life did the changing—I was the only thing changing! I told her I felt in some ways like my usefulness was over, that I'd worked so hard to love my family and do the things they needed for all these years. Now what was I to do?

She watched me as her knotty fingers began to gently pat out half the pastry dough into a circle on wax paper. Placing the dough into the dented aluminum pie plate and crimping the edges gently with her fingertips, she smiled at me.

"Why honey, you oughtn't to feel thatta way. You've raised your children to be good strong grown-ups with morals and values. You've made a home for your family and yo' life sure ain't over. Now you don't have to worry about such stuff as monthlies or having babies. That's not so bad now, is it?"

I sprinkled lemon juice over the apples and then stirred in cinnamon, nutmeg, and a bit of flour. Granny spooned them over the crust and began to pat out the second half of the dough. I put the pie in the oven to bake, then dropped ice cubes into two glasses and poured some iced tea.

Handing a glass to Granny, I sat back down. For close to an hour she listened as I poured out my heart and softly cried. All the while, the kitchen filled with the wonderful aroma of cinnamon and apples. I knew Granny understood, raising four children of her own and watching each leave home.

When the pie was done, Granny handed me a rose-flowered handkerchief from her apron pocket so I could dry my tears. She then spread a clean dishtowel on the countertop, removed the hot pie, and placed it on the counter to cool. She gazed out the window as she washed up the bowls and utensils and put them in the old wire dish drainer to dry.

I wondered what Granny was thinking, knowing she had a no-nonsense approach to life and plenty of country wisdom. I knew I had to wait and give her time to collect her thoughts. Granny couldn't be rushed.

"You know how much pride I take in my pies? I pour my love into them," she said. "Everyone loves my pies."

"Yes, Granny, of course."

"Well, life's not much different from making this here pie. You spend a lotta yo' time in life doing all that needs to be done, but then when you go through the change of life, well . . ."

She sliced a piece of the warm pie, piled a big scoop of vanilla bean ice cream on top and then gave it to me, along with a fork.

I waited for her to finish as the ice cream slowly trickled down. I took a bite of the warm, sweet pie—the taste of the tart apples and cinnamon and flaky crust was wonderful.

Still she didn't say anything, and as I looked into her kind, wrinkled eyes, I knew what she meant. I laughed out loud.

"Granny, it's like this pie. I've done the work and now it's time to eat!"

"Yes, honey." she smiled, "Now comes the good part!"

Kathy Reed

The Day I Joined the Club

A candle loses nothing by lighting another candle.

Father James Keller

When my fiancé, Kenny, and I arrived at the summer barbecue to celebrate our friend's birthday, I knew we would have a good time. I knew the food would be great. What I didn't know was that I would join a new club that day—the Hot Flash Club.

I'd been going through the early stages of menopause, quietly acknowledging that my periods had stopped and I was no longer a "woman of childbearing age." It was fairly early in my life, since I was only forty-three years old, just like my mom had been.

I had also been quietly suffering through the red, flushed face, beads of sweat, and the feeling that a furnace had been lit inside my body. It wasn't something I was proud of, and though I knew it was a common fact of life, I felt that I was alone in my circumstances.

And then, gathered in the home of the woman who was hosting our friend's party, it all changed.

Donna came in from her barbecuing duties outside, hair disheveled, face red, sweat beaded on her forehead and upper lip. "Now that's something every menopausal woman wants," she laughed. "It's no fun to stand over a barbecue on a July day while having a hot flash!" A few men looked on, puzzled. Some of the younger women smiled politely. But me, I laughed loud and hard. I made eye contact with this woman and with a couple of other forty- and fifty-something women nearby. We all laughed together. We shared the same picture, an image, a feeling that no one else in the group could relate to. It felt good!

It was then that I realized that I'd joined a new club, so to speak. I was part of a new group of women that I would identify with for the rest of my life. I had bonded with younger women before, not ignoring women older than myself, but certainly not spending much time thinking about them either.

Suddenly, these older women were *my* women. To me, our club motto could be summed up with the phrase, "I've lived." The goal of the club? To see what's next, to see what the rest of our lives will bring.

Today I look at women in their forties, fifties, sixties, and beyond. I see where I am now and where I am headed. I realize that I am certainly not alone in my menopausal experience. I have a certain "I-know-something-you-don't-know" feeling when I see women in their teens, twenties, and thirties. It is a "been there, done that" knowledge. Although I wouldn't have missed the early years for anything, I don't resent losing a portion of my youth.

But this is a new chapter, a new freedom. I still take care of myself, still talk with other women about clothes, men, and our careers. We have added talk about hair loss, vision changes, and what works best for aches and pains (not to mention those blasted hot flashes). The best thing is that nine times out of ten when I am talking to a fellow "club" member, we laugh about it. We know we can't change menopause, and we also know that in a way we are lucky to be experiencing it.

Club membership is free. And a sense of humor is mandatory.

Valerie Porter

A Thanksgiving Prayer

I wish they would only take me as I am.

Vincent van Gogh

"I hate Thanksgiving!" I moaned.

"You don't mean that," said my husband, Joe. He threw me a worried look as I grabbed my chef's knife and pointed it in his direction before I returned to chopping the celery in front of me.

"Yes, I do." I quickly grabbed an onion in hope of blaming the saltwater running down my cheeks on something other than my lousy frame of mind. While I knew I shouldn't let it, the mailman's morning delivery of another rejection letter for an article I'd submitted to a magazine made me feel like a black cloud of failure hung over my head.

Poor Joe. I never claimed to wear a halo, but he had had to run for cover more and more lately. I wiped my dripping forehead with the back of my free hand and fanned myself. I did loathe Thanksgiving, but there was a lot more going on here than rejections and a normal hissy fit. My doctor had warned me about mood swings, hot flashes, and sporadic periods. I knew the signs. It looked as if I'd officially entered menopause. This was it. Life was over. "I'm done with writing. I'll never get published," I moaned out loud. There, I'd admitted the fear I'd been carrying inside for months. "Fifty is too old."

Joe shook his head. "You're making too big a deal out of one rejection, the same way you're making too big a deal out of one holiday."

"You don't say. Well, if fighting crowds to shop, dragging bags stuffed with enough food to cause a hernia, and wrestling a slippery dead bird is so much fun, why don't men do it?" I bit my lip, aware that the words popping out of my mouth resembled ugly, poisonous toads.

"Some do. Ever heard of chefs?" my hubby grinned.

Joe and his logic!

"You need a break," he said. Keeping a careful eye on the position of my knife, he put his arms around me. "Go write something. I'll finish the chopping. Forget about what others want. Write for yourself. Count your blessings. Tell you what, why don't you write a special grace for tomorrow?"

"Fine," I handed him the knife, removed my apron, and fled the kitchen for my office. He wanted me to write grace? He'd get it!

"Feel better?" Joe asked when I entered the kitchen later. A mound of peeled potatoes bore witness that we'd both spent our time wisely.

"Actually, I do. I finished writing my idea of grace."

"Going to read it to me?"

"Tomorrow," I promised.

The next day I had to admit that my Thanksgiving table never looked better. The scent of that crispy brown turkey, fluffy mashed potatoes, savory stuffing, and assorted vegetables made even my mouth water. Joe clinked his spoon against his glass as everyone took their seats. "Michele's going to say grace."

Seated, I announced, "The Menopausal Woman's Thanksgiving Prayer." I stood up, trying to ignore the raised eyebrows from some of those present. "Dear God," I kept my eyes on the paper in front of me. "I'm thankful that having reached this period in life, I can now speak my mind and be considered wise, not obnoxious. I'm thankful that women my age will need bifocals to see the chin hairs that they missed plucking. I'm thankful that ninety-five percent of the stuff that I forget from here on will probably be unimportant anyway. I'm also thankful that Norman Rockwell painted his famous magazine cover with a perfect family and turkey as a model, not a rule of thumb." I smiled at Joe. "I'm also thankful for a husband who understands and loves me, even when I'm having a hard time accepting that I have to face this phase of aging. But, most of all, I'm thankful that the patience, strength, and fortitude that I've learned and developed as a young girl, wife, and mother has empowered me to never give up. Amen."

My family cheered as I sat down.

"Going to send that prayer out?" my husband whispered to me.

"Tomorrow," I replied.

And I did.

Michele H. Lacina

Menopause, Mommy, and Me

Experience is one thing you can't get for nothing.

Oscar Wilde

At family gatherings many years ago, "the change" was spoken of in hushed whispers among my aging aunts. While literally dozens of first, second, and third cousins whooped, hollered, ran, skipped, and rolled upon the sweet grass at Aunt Blanche's farm, many of the women fanned their red, perspiring faces with handkerchiefs, fans, or papers, whatever would generate a bit of refreshing breeze. Discreetly, they commiserated with each other.

Totally unsympathetic, we teenaged girls cast veiled, smug smirks at our older female relatives. Not one of us believed that we would become "mature." We were positive that we would always be young, firm-fleshed, and vibrant. At that time, anyone over the age of thirty had already passed into the nether regions of "old."

Time passed. Suddenly I was in my twenties, married, and the mother of a daughter and a son. I'm still not sure how it happened so quickly, but then overnight, I was in my late thirties, the mother of two teenagers. Ten more years galloped by, and something horrendous began going awry in my body.

The first night I awoke drenched in sweat, I thought that I had wet the bed! Horrors! Upon consideration, I realized that it was predominantly my head, neck, and upper body that were soaked. I changed my gown, turned over the pillow, punched it, and tried to go back to sleep, certain that some terrible disease was about to pounce upon me.

Over the course of the next two years, I had to admit that "the change" had taken over my life, and I didn't like it! On Sunday mornings I had refused to fan myself with the church bulletin until I saw other choir members do so. Unlike the Southern ladies who "glow," I didn't get dewy, or glow, or perspire. I would sweat! Rivulets ran down my cheeks, my neck, my back, and every other place where there was fabric that could stick to skin.

My daughter, who was close to thirty at that time, often teased me about my sudden red face, the beads of sweat above my upper lip, how I often pulled my blouse away from my body. "Just wait!" I told her, knowing that the menopause monster would attack her all too soon. I smiled at her. Except for a short period during her teens, she and I had always been good friends.

When she was a child, I often made matching dresses for both of us, real "mommy and me" garments, but that was before she was old enough to realize dressing like your mother wasn't cool. As adults, my daughter and I shared the same taste in clothing, furniture, and food. We have even chosen the same pieces of jewelry on separate shopping trips, and we often finish each other's sentences and answer questions at the same time using the same words.

At the age of fifty-five, I underwent a total hysterectomy. The ovarian tumor was benign, thankfully, and the doctor wanted me to start hormone replacement in the form of an estrogen patch. The majority of menopausal symptoms had disappeared, but he wanted me to benefit from all the other supposedly good things that hormone replacement offers. It was wonderful!

I faithfully applied a new little patch every week, except for a period of about a month when I kept forgetting to get the prescription refilled. When I told the druggist all of my old symptoms had returned, such as irritability, night sweats, hot flashes, and chills, he wanted to know how many people had sent me in to get the prescription filled!

All was well until early last autumn. At my biannual checkup, the doctor told me that I should discontinue using the patch; I had been wearing them for ten years, which was too long. "Let's see how you do," he said. Well, I didn't do well. Without the estrogen patch, I was drop-kicked back into the briar patch of full-blown menopause!

Then suddenly it dawned on me that my lovely daughter, who was now forty-five, had begun to fan, pull her blouse away from her body, use a sleeve, a napkin, a towel, a tablecloth, whatever fabric was available, to wipe her beautiful red face. We were sitting across from each other at a restaurant, both of us surreptitiously using a napkin to wipe sweat from our upper lips. Our eyes locked, and we both burst into laughter at the same time.

There we sat, the kindred spirit of menopause between us. Whoever would have thought that a mother and daughter, with twenty years difference in age, could share such a monumental experience? She was not yet to the stage that hormone replacement is recommended, but I had an edge. That very week I called my doctor and told him that I wanted my patch back.

He renewed the prescription, and I fully intend to continue wearing one of those little miracle workers for as long as I am able to slap it somewhere on my body. When the day comes that I am given my final bath, I can guarantee that the undertaker will find a little clear, oval patch on my abdomen or a hip, placed there tenderly by an arthritic hand—either mine *or* my husband's!

Barbara Elliott Carpenter

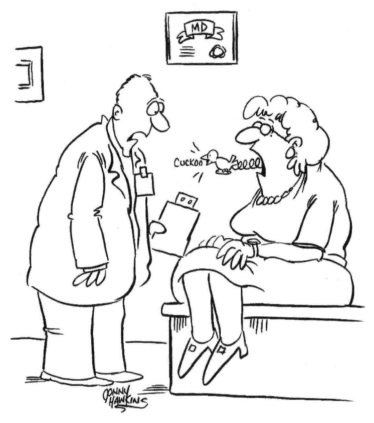

"There's something wrong with your body clock."

Wrinkled Anticipation

Where there is great love, there are always wishes.

Willa Cather

I opened my eyes one wink at a time, stretched, rolled over, and stared at the body lying next to me. *Was it breathing?* I thought. I stared for a long time. Yes, its chest rose and fell in adagio. Sleeping Beauty was blissfully at rest and completely unaware of my desires. *Silly me, why did I expect today to be any different?*

Yawning away the last remnants of sleep as sunbeams glimmered into view, I prepared to embrace this special day to its fullest. I planned to start it off with Vivaldi's *Spring* playing in the background while I ate breakfast in bed: eggs Benedict, a mimosa, an Italian pastry, and an espresso with anisette to top it off. Yum! Willing to risk the hot flashes that alcohol ignites these days, I salivated at the thought. *Surely, my fifty-fifth birthday merited such celebratory self-indulgence!*

I got up without making a sound, slid into my slippers, and wrestled into my robe. I refused to wash sleep's patina off my face, reserving the right to return to bed later and doze away the warming sunshine. Ambling into my office, I switched on the computer. *Maybe I shouldn't give up hope,* I thought. *An animated e-card might await me with a birthday greeting and special itinerary for today.* I hoped for any kind of acknowledgment, but received none.

A half hour later Sleeping Beauty sauntered into the office, looked at me for a long minute, groaned, stretched, and tottered off into the kitchen. Not even a happy birthday kiss. As usual, I prepared breakfast for both of us. I settled for cottage cheese with cinnamon and a cup of decaffeinated coffee, while the object of my affection ate cereal and drank plain tap water—but not very mannerly. Those slurping sounds and the cereal spilling onto the floor made me cringe more than usual today, but I tolerated it for love.

I'm not ashamed to admit that I'm much older than Sleeping Beauty, or that we moved in together after only one date—just a few days before Christmas, six weeks ago. The holiday wasn't much fun, though. Sleeping Beauty took a spill while trying to scale a fence and spent Christmas Eve in the hospital under observation for a concussion. I played nursemaid on Christmas Day, doing all I could to make my patient comfortable; I put pillows and blankets on the sofa next to our Christmas tree and played Christmas carols in the background for ambience. My dizzied patient hugged me, kissed me, and made other loving gestures—but there was no package for me to unwrap. Don't get me wrong; after twenty years without this kind of affection, those loving gestures were dear to me, but still, I felt a twinge of neglect. And then I felt guilty about feeling neglected. So, while I lavished gifts on my new squeeze, I pretended that the absence of a material expression of love didn't bother me. That was the beginning of our affair—and the harbinger of my current plight.

I'm the kind of person who has to work hard at being

carefree and spontaneous, and as you might expect, my new love is just the opposite. Sharing my life with Sleeping Beauty gives me a newfound freedom; we play a lot and do things on impulse. But I bear all responsibility for our lifestyle. I make many accommodations for Sleeping Beauty's devil-may-care attitude, too, especially in sharing my home. I never expected to find things strewn all over, or to continually pick up and clean up after my love.

What compels me to make so many sacrifices for so little in return? It isn't good looks—that long, pointy nose and those big ears are not your typical heart-throb attributes (although admirers of Cyrano de Bergerac and Clark Gable might disagree). Perhaps it's those titillating feelings I get from those soft, wet kisses, long embraces and cuddling on the loveseat. Or maybe it's the frolicking and playfulness that makes me feel like I did back in the days before arthritis barnacled my bones. Menopause didn't shut everything down! Today is a good day to reflect. During this morning's early hours, I crossed a threshold; I'm no kid anymore. Yet, despite the supposed wisdom of my age, I expected things to suddenly be different. Love can be blinding, even to the oldest and wisest among us.

We didn't go back to bed. I felt the sunlight heat up and cool again as I fed and picked up after Sleeping Beauty between heavy petting sessions. Still, I wouldn't let go of my fantasy that a surprise might be in store for me. All day, I expected flowers to arrive at any moment. I jumped every time a doorbell rang on a television show. I even fantasized that the card attached to the flowers would announce dinner reservations at a fine restaurant. I wanted to be Sleeping Beauty on my birthday—awakened by my Prince Charming into a life of doting, affection, and luxury!

When no sign of celebration manifested by early

evening I bargained with myself. *Why couldn't I just be happy with love and affection? Why did I want more? When did I become so materialistic?* I tried to convince myself that I should be happier.

As I accepted responsibility for my choices and trade-offs, the noise in my head quieted. Then, just as I surrendered to the lackluster quality of the day, my fantasy came true! My husband came home from work with flowers and exquisite dinner plans!

I put Sleeping Beauty in her kennel. Menopausal women cannot live on puppy love alone.

Marilyn Haight

Living with a Woman Possessed

Sometimes the heart sees what is invisible to the eye.

H. Jackson Brown, Jr.

My mother was always a sane, rational person who was able to control herself in any situation. All of that was altered during "the change," as menopause was called in earlier days. During that time, my dear, sweet, dependable mother was possessed by some evil force that invaded not only her body, but her mind and soul as well.

Mother suffered through the anguish brought on by a menstrual cycle. Without knowing exactly the cause, we three boys (my older brother and my twin and I) knew to keep low profiles about the same time each month. During those few days, this woman, who was our strength after our dad died in 1965, seemed a bit more fatigued. She often came home from a day of teaching sixth grade and dropped her tired body onto the couch.

"I need just ten minutes of rest before I start supper." And with that, Mother fell asleep for at most half an hour. Then she was up and about her regular duties.

We also knew that she sometimes had stomach cramps,

and at times they completely doubled her over. She always told us boys not to worry, and she toughed her way through those gut-wrenching episodes. I never saw her swallow an aspirin or a Midol to help ease the pain of her period. She was from that generation that didn't believe in taking medicine to alleviate what were small hurts. Neither did she use PMS as an excuse for letting herself fly out of control.

All of that strong side took a hiatus for her time of menopause. During those years, life was especially touchy around our house. My mother was a warm-natured woman to begin with, so the hot flashes that she endured must have made her feel that she was living in the fiery pit of hell. We had no air conditioning in the house, so her only relief was a window fan. Many nights Mother walked the floor in fits of insomnia that were often brought on by those surging temperatures in her body.

A later condition at least partially attributable to menopause was the increasing fragility of her bones. A woman who had spent her life enjoying manual labor in the yard and at jobs before she became a teacher broke both of her wrists within a few years.

The most frightening aspect of Mother's journey through menopause concerned her mood swings. She'd always been a stern, no-nonsense kind of parent. Simply put, rules were established, and she expected us boys to abide by them. As she experienced the forces of a hateful invader that comes with age, she often acted as one who had fallen under evil influences. One particular episode remained with us over the years.

On Saturday mornings, we three boys were to clean the house. That meant vacuuming and dusting every room, as well as cleaning sinks, toilets, and closets. Mother fixed pancakes or waffles on those weekend mornings, and we watched cartoon shows and *American Bandstand* before beginning our work. One Saturday morning, Mother decided that we needed to begin cleaning early. She called to us to begin; in fact, she called twice. After we failed to respond, she squalled like an angry wildcat, "You boys get busy right NOW!" We recognized the change in her voice, but again tempting fate, we returned to the programs on the television.

A few minutes later, I rose and walked into the hall to assemble the vacuum. At that very moment, a jar whizzed by my head and shattered on the door leading to the basement. As I tried to stop my heart from racing and regain my composure, Mother appeared at the other end of the hall. Although she was only five feet, two inches tall, she appeared at that moment to be gigantic. Her eyes shot fire, and my brothers and I knew that she was in the grips of "the change" and that our only way of escaping more ire was to complete our work quickly and quietly.

In later years we boys laughed about the incident., However, Mother always countered, "I never did any such thing." We had grown into men who had married, and by then, we'd become authorities on the terrible things through which women go. Mother had truly been possessed by the brutal forces of menopause; however, on the other side of the change, we found the same wonderful woman who had always loved us and had given so much of herself to our well-being. Receiving all that love made those difficult times seem rather insignificant.

Joe Rector

Take a Midlife Chance

*One's mind, once stretched by a new idea,
never regains its original dimensions.*

Oliver Wendell Holmes

My husband, Scott, dreamed of owning a motorcycle again, like the one he owned as a teenager back in 1974—those weekends when he tore up neighbors' yards, using his parents' lawnmower gas to fuel his bike. I rolled my eyes and said, "Yeah, like that will ever happen." I caught a slight look of hurt shoot across his face and felt a slight twinge of guilt, because I usually got what I wanted, including his undying support for my ideas and many career changes over our twenty years together. *He must be going through his midlife crisis,* I reasoned to myself. Of course, I wasn't; at age forty-something, I knew who I was, and I didn't need some dangerous toy to make me feel young again.

My national tea flavoring company had really been flourishing, due in part to his creative mind and support. Scott had listened to my endless chatter on ideas for tea blends, logo designs, and distributor issues. He sacrificed many hours helping my company grow, along with his regular full-time job as a custom home builder. Finally, out of sheer guilt, I relented, and the happy man got his wish. After balancing the books and doing a bit of juggling, I called him at work and found myself uttering those dreaded words: "Maybe you should pick out a motorcycle. I think we can swing it." I immediately heard the phone drop and the wild scampering of feet off to the dealership.

Soon there was a shiny new black Honda VTX 1300 in our driveway and a very happy man grinning from ear to ear standing alongside it. The men in the neighborhood gathered around, as if gazing at a scantily clad supermodel washing a car. The testosterone was so thick I almost grew chest hair myself. My happy man was the envy of the cul-de-sac.

Then I began to hear a question I had never contemplated having to answer. "Honey, please go for a ride with me? Just try it once," he begged.

"Not a chance, never!" I repeated each time. I justified this by reminding myself that I would be his first passenger in three decades. I imagined myself lying on the road, bugs plastered on my teeth, helmet hair, and a whole slew of related horrors flashing in my mind's eye.

Days went by and I noticed such a change in Scott's demeanor. He was not just a happy little camper, he was full of *joy*. He smiled a Cheshire cat grin when wearing his helmet, sometimes even wearing it around the kitchen. He reminded me of my son with his first Big Wheel. Scott was gone for hours, alone, riding until dusk. He came home after his rides, relaxed and peaceful.

Secretly, I wanted to see what this was all about, without giving him the satisfaction of my curiosity. After years of scolding him for wanting a dangerous frivolous toy, how could I? I begged the question inside, *Why did this dangerous fancy bicycle on steroids make him so relaxed?* Is a whole generation of women wrong to pay someone to rub our backs, paint our toenails, and bend us into impossible positions in yoga classes all in the name of stress reduction? Have our male counterparts held the secret all along? Eat pork rinds over the sink, watch television, drink out of the milk carton, hop on a bike, and be fulfilled? Most women I knew were popping Prozac from a Pez dispenser, running from class to class in search of the answer.

Don't ask me how, but weeks later I found myself allowing Scott to tuck my hair into a helmet as I got ready to ride. Yes, you heard me, *ride*. With an excited grin on his face, he went over the "rules," a crash course on how to sit and how to lean into each turn. "Like a dance," he said, "let me lead, honey." The word shot through me. Let him *lead?* I began to panic . . . I never let anyone lead! I groaned inside as I climbed aboard, hoping the neighbors weren't looking, since I had publicly announced several times, "I will never get on that thing."

I felt my heart race as the ground sped by at what seemed like 100 miles an hour. I yelled over the roar of the wind, rather angrily in fact, for him to "slow it down already." Feeling silly as he pointed to the speedometer, whose tiny needle was hardly at 10 mph, I slumped back. I had to trust him. After all, only God knew when my number was up; I really couldn't control that, right? Plus, I was wearing clean underwear, and my hair was recently highlighted and cut, so if I was going to go, now would be as good a time as any. *I might as well enjoy it,* I reasoned. Snuggling into his warm leather jacket, I looked ahead over his shoulder like a child on a carnival ride.

It's funny what you experience when you let someone else take you away to their private joy, to their own slice of heaven, and not insist on always being in control of your own pastimes, your own comfort zones, your own daily grind. Shamefully, I soon realized how selfish I had become. This was his dream, and he wanted to share it with *me*. Not his friends—those envious driveway buddies—but me. I felt the guilt consume me, and the shame of finding out what I had been missing all along. All the passed up opportunities in my life flashed back to me, all the resounding "Not this time, thanks." The memories I stole from myself out of selfishness and stubborn unwillingness to bend, evolve, and share with someone else. I realized that I was the one in the midlife crisis, a crisis of being stuck somewhere between older and dead.

Now I know that joy can be found in many things, including other people's things, even in my man's world of little boy stuff. From now on I will take chances; I don't ever want to be in a midlife crisis again. I want to grow as I grow old.

Lisa Wynn

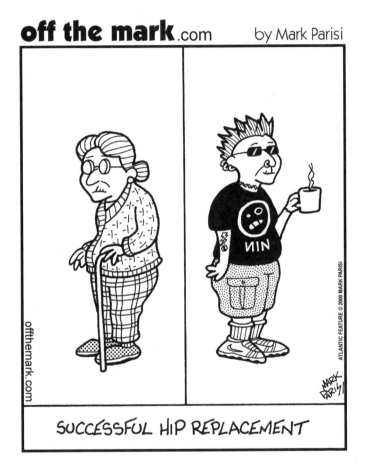

Mom and the Menopause Booth

A mother is she who can take the place of all others, but whose place no one else can take.

Cardinal Mermillod

To promote my first book about menopause, I attended a women's show in St. Louis. Unfortunately, the frigid February winds turned the expected throng of attendees into a trickle, and a major snowstorm closed the show a day early. The weekend could have been considered a dud, but it became one of my better memories, because I shared that weekend with my mom.

Under normal circumstances, one of my sisters would have accompanied me on a trip like this, but Sister One was out of town on a work assignment, and Sister Two had two small sons who needed her at home. My hubby offered to come, but the thought of a man at a women's gathering—in a menopause booth—wasn't too practical. Several of my girlfriends said they would go, but spending a weekend with friends is a good way to lose friends, so that was out, too.

Mom had also volunteered to come with me. In fact, she

had been the first to volunteer, but I was afraid her arthritis would make navigating the huge St. Louis Convention Center nearly impossible. She insisted. So we loaded her wheelchair into the van next to a dozen boxes of books, and headed east to St. Louis.

Some women may shudder at the thought of spending a weekend with their mom, but not me. My mom has always been one of my best buddies. I looked forward to spending time with her. In 1999, Mom found a lump in her breast that turned out to be malignant. The doctor thought surgery had removed the cancer, but in 2002 we learned it had returned. Although it was a very slow growing cancer, it had metastasized to Mom's liver and lungs. So you understand why I cherish every moment I can spend her.

Besides that, Mom's a hoot. Everyone loves her. Vendors in nearby booths were soon calling her "Mom" and stopping by to chat. When the crowd was slow, Mom would head off in her wheelchair, foot-powered like Fred Flintstone. She'd return twenty minutes later with a lap full of vendor freebies—booklets, pens, bottled water, toiletry samples, munchies, plastic sacks, and even a clock!

Our customers loved Mom, too. Although it was blustery outside, one lady passed the booth with beads of sweat literally rolling off her forehead. "Hot flash?" Mom asked, extending a box of pink tissues to the woman. The woman swabbed her face. "Even my hair is wet," she moaned, fluffing the moist hair along her hairline. "Here, honey. I'll give you the whole box if you buy one of my daughter's books." The sweaty lady bought two and left our booth dabbing happy-tears and a drippy forehead with her newly acquired box of pink tissues.

The women who really connected with my mom were the ones who wanted to talk about hormones and breast cancer. Mom wanted to learn about their cancer experiences. At those times, she wasn't merely my mother; she was a woman with a need to learn more about the frightening invader in her body.

It's been three years since our St. Louis excursion. Mom's cancer has slowly spread into her bones and brain, but she's spunky as ever. We often reminisce about our St. Louis excursion: How we giggled at the woman who bragged she had never had even one menopausal symptom, apparently unaware of the forest of curly hairs dangling from her chin! How we backed off and raised eyebrows when grumpy women vehemently denied they were menopausal. Of course, it didn't help that their friends nudged them in the ribs, pointed to our booth and said, "That's what you need—a book about menopause. Har-har!"

Mom still chuckles about the lady who swung around suddenly, flipping her blonde wig off her head and onto the floor! The gal scooped it up, plopped it back over her messy mop of real hair, and waltzed off like nothing happened. Back in the hotel room after a ten-hour day, Mom and I propped ourselves up in our queen-sized beds and ate popcorn and leftover Italian food and talked. We didn't sleep much, though, because neither of us could muffle the other's snoring, even with earplugs!

Without a doubt, that was a wild and crazy weekend, but I wouldn't have changed a thing. I will always cherish those memories of Mom with me at the menopause booth.

Donna Rogers

EDITOR'S NOTE: Donna's mother, Mary DeShon, passed away peacefully on December 4, 2006. She was seventy-five years young. Mary was excited that Donna had submitted "their" menopausal story, and even though she would never see it in print, Mary was extremely proud of her daughter.

Pass the Peas, Please

"Pass the peas, honey," my husband said. "Dinner is great, by the way."

Noticeably suppressing a giggle, I picked up the bowl and handed it to him. "Did I say something amusing?" he asked. I smiled in return.

"Oh no, I was just thinking . . . well, er . . . I'm just pleased you like the meal." I popped a forkful of peas into my mouth, savoring both the taste and the recent memory.

The evening before I was at one of the "ladies only" gatherings at the ranch where I boarded my horse. We started having potlucks with a few of us who just happened to be in that range of womanhood I like to call the "power years," somewhere between forty-five and sixty-five. We were all at the pre-, present, or post-menopausal phases of our lives and "power surges" (aka hot flashes) were familiar, albeit unwelcome, visitors.

Relaxed and satiated after a great dinner and some good wine, we were ready for dessert on the back deck. It usually included chocolate in some form, and one of us brought all the fixings to make s'mores on the open barbecue. The aroma of melting chocolate and marshmallow was pure heaven, and we salivated while cooking our individual creations to the perfect degree of gooeyness.

I was licking my fingers after my first s'more and contemplating another when Liz suddenly sprang from her chair howling, "Oh God, I'm burning up!"

I gasped and jumped up, thinking she had caught her clothes on fire. Upon closer inspection, I could see what she was dealing with. Bright splotchy red patches from her hairline down her neck and onto her chest revealed a doozy of a hot flash.

"They're driving me crazy, I can't stand this!" Liz moaned. I could feel a lump in my throat as I remembered the discomfort of similar times. Diane jumped up and started fanning Liz with a paper plate; Jan handed her a glass of water. I ran to the freezer to get an ice pack and, finding none, I grabbed the next best thing—a bag of frozen peas. I ran back to Liz and slapped the bag of peas on the back of her neck. Not knowing that it was peas on her neck, Liz sighed, "That feels so-o-o good. Do you have another?" I ran back and found a bag of frozen corn and brought that out to place on her chest. When Liz and the other women realized what I had actually done, they erupted into gales of laughter. That brought on a mini hot flash for Di, so I ran back and brought out whatever frozen vegetables I could find and passed them around.

Through tears of laughter, Jill gasped, "You've thawed out most of my frozen veggies on your hot bodies. Now what am I going to do with them?"

Some little evil part of me responded with, "Hey, let's each take a bag home and feed them to our husbands tomorrow. They'll never know the difference. It'll be our little secret." They all agreed. The next evening I made a special dinner of pot roast, potatoes, carrots, salad, and, you guessed it, beautiful "flash-cooked" green peas, my husband's favorite. Bon appétit!

I wonder what Liz served her husband? She was making humorous hints about keeping some frozen Hershey bars on hand for the next big flash and trying that instead of veggies because she likes chocolate better. Come to think of it, so might her husband. Hmmmmm.

Linda Leary

5

IN THE NAME
OF LOVE

Love builds bridges where there are none.

R.H. Delaney

A Dose of Reality

Perimenopause was beginning to frustrate me to no end. From sagging body parts to fledging chin hairs, from fading eyesight to a fading memory, getting use to this phase of my life at age forty-three was slowly becoming a reality. But no one could make this fact more evident to me than my ten-year-old son, Shawn.

From the day he was born, Shawn has always been on the small side. To keep up his self-esteem, the family has always made it a point to praise him for growing taller, using everyday household objects to gauge his growth. From the first time Shawn was able to see in the bathroom mirror by himself without having to use a stool, to being able to sit at the family dinner table without a telephone book, growth milestones in Shawn's life have been a constant in our home.

One favorite growth milestone for Shawn was the kitchen countertop. When he had grown tall enough to finally see over the counter, we had to come up with another growth milestone. Looking around the house, the next obvious one was growing tall enough to see over the top of the refrigerator; at five-foot, seven-inches tall, I couldn't even see over the top of this large appliance.

Stumped, we finally agreed to measure him to me, deciding to use my boobs as his new growth milestone.

One of my favorite things in the world is to get hugs from my boy, who is very lovable, caring, and compassionate. Whenever he would hug me, I'd say, "Oh, Shawn, you're almost as tall as my boobs!" He'd just laughed, mainly because I would say the word "boobs" to him.

Then reality set in. One morning, when I was enjoying my wake-up hug from Shawn, I was shocked by how tall he was compared with my boobs. It was as if he had grown four inches overnight!

"Shawn, look how tall you are! You're taller than my boobs," I exclaimed to him, mid-hug.

Shawn pulled away and looked up at me with sleepy eyes. He mumbled, "Duh, Mom. You're not wearing a bra." He then walked into the living room to play his Game Cube.

I stood in the kitchen, dumbfounded. Looking down at my perimenopausal body, I realized that Shawn hadn't grown four inches overnight, but quite the opposite; my boobs had decided to sag four inches. With no chance of a boob job in the immediate future, we still have yet to find another growth milestone for my loving, compassionate, caring, and honest ten-year-old!

Dahlynn McKowen

Hey, Baby

Woman begins by resisting a man's advances and ends by blocking his retreat.

Oscar Wilde

I was waiting in line at the gas station when a truck pulled out from the other side of the island. As it passed my car, the driver, who must have been in his late thirties, if that, leaned out of the open window and said, "Hey, baby," directly to me. Then he grinned, eased his truck into traffic, and disappeared.

Time stopped dead in its radial-tired, all-wheel-drive tracks as I processed what had just happened. My first thought was that the man shouldn't be on the road because obviously he had a vision problem. Then I wondered if he was making fun of me, giving a thrill to the little old lady in the sporty Honda. Maybe he had a thing for older women? Or perhaps it was a random act of kindness, in a macho sort of way. My feminist indignation flared only to be squelched by my girlish delight. After all, I hadn't been whistled at or made the object of a sexist remark in many-a-year.

Was it possible that I could still be a "baby?"

The question stayed in my mind for the rest of the day. It followed me into the supermarket, inserting itself into the produce aisle between the broccoli and red leaf lettuce. It interrupted my thoughts when I was writing, and it came out in the middle of a scene for my latest children's story when all I wanted to attend to was how to get my main character out of the clutches of the schoolyard bully. "Go away," I told it. But the question remained. Was it possible, in my late fifties, to think of myself as a "baby"?

This was annoying me. My feminist roots bristled at the idea that I was even thinking about this for more than a nanosecond. Who cared what some guy in a truck rudely called out?

But it wasn't that, not really. What I was grappling with was my own sense of self. Did I feel like a "baby"? I used to. I used to know that my body was alluring, that my walk was confident. My smile used to be inviting. When I talked, people were drawn to me and my conversation. I had a sense of myself. Was I connected to my sensuality anymore? To myself?

That truck driver didn't know what he had stirred up. As I simmered the soup for dinner, I took stock of my life. What I saw was an accomplished, creative, strong woman with many friends and a wonderful family. Some days I felt more desirable than others, but that hadn't changed as I matured. What I realized was that I am a "baby" as much as I choose to be. When I am loving within myself, it shines and is attractive to others.

My husband came home in the middle of these thoughts. His eyes lit up when he saw me, and he said, "Hi, baby."

I wrapped my arms around him and silently sent a thank-you to the driver who recognized the "baby" in me when I had almost forgotten her.

Ferida Wolff

Sweet Advice

If you're a husband and you return home to find your wife sitting with no clothes on, her feet in a bucket of ice, and fanning herself, please be careful about your reaction.

You could say any of the following:

DANGEROUS: "WHAT in the WORLD are you DOING?"
SAFER: "You look nice and cool, dear!"
SAFEST: "I have always loved your birthday suit!"
or ULTRA-SAFE: "Here, have some chocolate!"

And if your wife seems a bit "off the wall" due to a hormonal imbalance, you could choose any of the following reactions:

DANGEROUS: "I don't know why you're so worked up!"
SAFER: "Could you be overreacting?"
SAFEST: "Here's the credit card, honey."
or ULTRA-SAFE: "Here, have some chocolate!"

Beverly Walker

Mom Must Be Dying

Nothing in life is to be feared, it is only to be understood.

Marie Curie

My sister Dana whispered to me, "Gigi, Mom's dying, and they don't want us to know." We were in the hallway trying to be as quiet as two teenage girls could be.

I whispered back, "That must be it. I thought Mom was going crazy. Maybe she has an inoperable brain tumor?" I continued on with my diagnosis, "That must be why she hasn't been to the doctor. There's nothing to be done." Tears filled our eyes.

Still whispering, Dana replied, "Mom has been acting strangely: She forgets everything we tell her, she has no patience, and do you see how much she sweats?"

Mom yelled from the living room, "You girls need to stop what you're doing if it requires you to whisper!"

Making our way into Dana's room, I plopped on her bed in frustration. I had more news to share with her.

"You won't believe what Mom forgot, Dana. She was so upset because she had to go back to the store. She went to buy some last-minute items for dinner and forgot them. She said she was distracted because she didn't want to forget to pick up the dry cleaning!"

Dana replied, "How can you forget the groceries when you only had two errands to remember?" It confirmed to us that her memory loss was getting worse.

Over the next few months my sister and I continued to worry. Mom had good days where she acted like her normal self, followed by bad days when nothing we did was right. She had a very short fuse, and her patience level seemed nonexistent. We resolved to have a bit more patience with her—we didn't want to be any trouble. Mom carried a hand towel to wipe the sweat that dripped from her face, and she also had trouble remembering our conversations. We both tried to ignore her obviously embarrassing sweating episodes and offered to help fill in the blanks when she forgot what she was about to say midsentence.

Dad was clueless. It was obvious that something was wrong with Mom, but he chose to ignore it all. He walked around the house shaking his head and murmuring to himself, "Oh my goodness." This was a bit puzzling to us; why wasn't he taking Mom to the doctor? Couldn't he see how sick she was?

One day after school, I stared in amazement as my mom began to sweat while watching television. The sweat ran down her beet-red face, and her shirt soaked up the moisture as she desperately fanned herself and wiped the sweat with a towel. It was probably bad timing to remind her that I was supposed to go to my friend's house to work on a class project and we had planned on meeting at 4:00 PM. I gathered my books and the materials I needed to bring with me, but when I told her that it was time to leave, she said that I couldn't go because she didn't know about it!

I yelled in frustration, "Mom, what is wrong with you?" Teary eyed, as she often was, she turned a darker shade of red—which I didn't think was humanly possible—and shouted at the top of her voice, "I'm going through menopause!"

I had no idea what menopause was (this was long before HRT, wild yam creams, natural estrogen pills, or the oh-so-helpful prescription drug commercials), so I asked her. She explained, in the same short cryptic dialogue she used when she gave me "the talk," that when a woman reaches a certain age her monthly cycle stops. Because of this, hormones can fluctuate during that time, resulting in hot flashes, mood swings, and memory difficulties. *No brain tumor,* I thought. I was relieved. I could hardly wait to tell Dana that Mom wasn't going insane or dying!

As we were driving to my friend's house, I asked Mom, "How long does it take to get through menopause?"

When my Mom finally stopped laughing, she wiped her brow and replied, "You don't want to know."

Genevra Bonati

A Husband's Love

Every problem has a gift for you in its hands.

Richard Bach

When I entered menopause, I opted not to have hormone replacement because of the cancer and heart disease risks that ran in my family. So I went cold turkey, and it was tough, in spite of my trying a variety of homeopathic remedies.

On one memorable night, I was tossing and turning in bed, unable to get comfortable. I had been averaging two to four hours of sleep a night. I'd wake up several times drenched with perspiration and needing to change nightgowns. Then I would have trouble getting back to sleep no matter how tired I was. On this one night, I couldn't fall asleep at all and was so restless that I woke up my husband.

"Honey, what can I do for you?" he asked sleepily.

"Nothing," I said. "It's just so terribly hot in here."

"It's not hot. If anything, it's very cold."

I realized that I'd pulled the covers off both of us and that he must be freezing.

"Sorry, my thermostat is on the blink again."

"How about if I bring up some ice water for you?"

"Thanks," I said.

After I'd cooled off a bit, I tried again to rest, but I still felt restless. My husband, as usual, was sensitive to my discomfort.

"Want me to turn on the television or the radio?"

"No thanks. Maybe I should go downstairs and try to read for a while."

"Not a good idea," he said.

"Why not?"

"You have to work in the morning," he said, adding, "I've got a better idea. Want to snuggle?"

"I do, but I can't stand to have anything warm against my skin right now."

He let out a deep sigh. "Are you sure? I think it's the best cure for anything that ails you."

"I'll go down for chamomile tea," I said.

"Honey, you do what you want." I could tell he was getting irritated himself.

"Hey, I'm the one who's suffering here," I said, becoming edgy.

"You know how I used to get nauseated right along with you when you were pregnant, and how I even felt your pain when your back hurt?"

"Yes," I said, remembering his sympathetic symptoms with a smile.

"Remember all the tofu recipes I've been agreeing to let you try out, and me not even liking the stuff?"

"Sure. You've been great," I conceded.

"Well, honey, right now, I'm just plain out of patience. I have to work tomorrow too, and I'm really tired." With that, he took his pillow and went into one of the other bedrooms. Both our sons were away at college, so there was plenty of space to spread out. I felt truly bereft.

I went downstairs, had my tea and a slice of dry toast, read a mystery novel for a little while, and then finally went back to bed. I still tossed and turned. I moved from my side of the bed to my husband's side, but I just couldn't get comfortable.

Finally, my husband returned to our bedroom.

"I thought you'd gone to sleep," I said.

"I heard you moving around. Come on, let's give the snuggling a try," he said. "For my sake, if not for yours."

I moved into his arms, and we kissed, and then we snuggled. He made me forget all about menopause. And after a time, we both slept peacefully and soundly.

Jacqueline Seewald

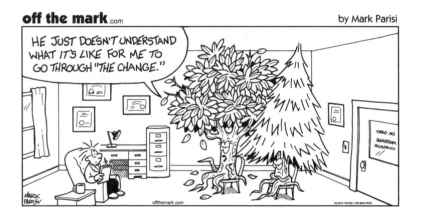

Reprinted by permission of Off the Mark and Mark Parisi. ©1996 Mark Parisi.

License to Complain

Trust yourself; you know more than you think you do.

Dr. Benjamin Spock

I was having an emotional meltdown and pity party. Wasn't it bad enough just to grow older, besides having to deal with menopause and its symptoms every day? I wanted to know why I had to grow facial hair and inflate each month like a helium balloon.

But menopause was small compared with the real source of my uncertainty. Sitting in a Best Western Inn in Mississippi 24/7 for six weeks was adding to my anxiety and misery. My husband's company had merged once again, and if he wanted to keep his position on the sales force, we had to move from our beautiful new Kentucky dream home. I was stunned. We had only lived there six months, and I wasn't finished doing the window treatments yet. I loved our home and being a part of the local Welcome Wagon with other wives. I felt so much a part of our community.

The only positive thing about the move was that only

three of our five children would have to experience this upheaval (my husband's two oldest children were married). My seventeen-year-old son Chris had been on the varsity basketball team and dreamed of going to state his senior year with the team. Jason, my husband's fifteen-year-old son, had to leave behind a girlfriend who did so much to boost his self-confidence. And Anne, my fourteen-year-old daughter, was happy at school; as a freshman, she was ingrained with a group of girls who shared the scoop on every neat guy and liked the same music, often going to concerts together when big-named stars came to Louisville.

Having always been enrolled in public school up to this point, our three teenagers were now going to attend Pillow Academy, a small private school established in 1962 during the desegregation conflict. I thought I was well aware of the losses my teenagers were feeling, and I worried about their acceptance at Pillow Academy. All the students had their own cars to drive to school; school buses were simply not practical since the students came from such a large area that represented more than one school district. I only had to look at the school parking lot full of BMWs, Volvos, and new trucks to know that the student body was far from poor. My three teenagers were appalled to have me drive them to school each day like the mothers of grade school children do. Since we were living in the Best Western and not on a cotton plantation, I thought the least I could do was let my son take the car and give the kids some dignity. Even at that, they were somewhat embarrassed. They nicknamed my big four-door Mercury the "Land Barge."

It wasn't long until I started meeting other mothers at school events. Wow! They all looked like retired Miss America contestants. They were slim and some were active in tennis, going to tournaments often over the weekends in other states. They played bridge and had "help" to do the housework, yard work, and ironing. Since I did not play tennis or bridge, my opportunity to socialize in their groups was limited.

While my husband was busy traveling the state, calling on cotton farmers to sell an insecticide that would kill boll weevils, I was looking at houses with a local realtor. We wanted to find a four-bedroom house to rent, where each of the kids could have their own room like they had enjoyed in Kentucky. Discouraged after a day of looking at homes that were dismal and dumpy, I plopped onto the hotel room bed, staring into space.

Soon, the kids came home from school; Jason and Anne immediately donned their swimming suits and headed to the hotel's heated indoor pool. Chris stayed with me. He was only four years old when his father and I divorced. Even as a little boy, he was aware of the void in my life and felt responsible to fill it. Chris would always ask me, "Momma, are you happy? Are you sad?" Then he would do somersaults to make me laugh or give me reassuring hugs and kisses that everything would be okay.

Doing what was natural to him, Chris asked me his two standard questions that afternoon. I don't know why I couldn't be honest with him and just say that I was having a real hard time fitting in here. My kids liked Pillow Academy and their new friends. Their dad was enjoying talking with the plantation owners and seeing the country. I, on the other hand, was stuck in a hotel room, feeling fat, unathletic, and unattractive. That would have been too simple to just tell Chris, I guess. But I was raging inside with frustration, aided by my menopause. The next thing I knew, these horrible words were spewing out of my mouth: "Chris, if there is such a thing as reincarnation, I hope you come back to the next life as a woman so you can know what it feels like to have cramps, a bloated stomach, and painful breasts. I am not having a good day!"

He looked at me with sad eyes and said in a voice that was kind but searing, "Well, Mom, if there is such a thing as reincarnation, I hope that you come back to the next life as a child of divorced parents so you will know what it is like to have every Christmas, birthday, and Thanksgiving feel like one parent you love is missing, no matter which parent you're with. You will get to know what it is like to wonder what the other parent is doing and if they are happy or sad without you."

He turned and left the room. I was horrified to think that I had blasted him in a menopausal moment. Why did I think that menopause gave me a license to complain? Why had I spoken so bluntly? I felt I deserved his retort, and I never mentioned it to him again. I did learn that those suffering in silence may have daily pain or agony that they endure, but not every ache and pain needs to be shared with family and friends.

Today my son is a wonderful, loving husband and father. He still calls me from Chicago to see how I am doing, always asking, "Momma, are you happy? Are you sad?" I make sure my answers aren't chronic complaints, only answers of love and acceptance.

Linda H. Puckett

God, I'm Shvitzing!

"So, what did the doctor say?" I asked as I entered our bedroom.

My wife, Lisa, reached over and gave me a soft "welcome home" kiss. I could tell the news was not going to be good. "He saw signs I may be going through perimenopause."

"Perimenopause?" I asked. I knew about menopause, but what the heck was perimenopause? Noting the confusion on my face and in my voice, she immediately answered, "It marks the period that begins the transition into menopause."

I learned from her that perimenopause symptoms vary from woman to woman; however, they can include hot flashes, menstrual irregularities, loss of sexual arousal, sleeping problems, and, of course, mood swings. When she told me that this could last anywhere from two to eight years, in addition to the actual menopause period, chills went up my spine.

"Eight years!"

"Yeah," she replied. The unspoken sadness in her voice was louder than any of her words. She would soon be entering what is commonly known as the "change of life." She was barely in her forties.

"Eight years," I repeated in disbelief. "You've got to be kidding!"

She wasn't, and it was a stupid question, even for a rhetorical one. I was going to enter somewhat of a change of life, too. And as hard as I tried to resist, my mind visualized the various clichéd situations I had seen in numerous movies and television shows. But reality would soon alter my perspective.

Yes, the mood swings were touchy, but I soon got accustomed to them and tried not to take them personally. Sometimes this was not an easy task.

Yes, the lowered libido was troublesome. But like the famous car rental service, that meant we just had to work harder, but with care.

But the hot flashes. This was what made my heart truly ache for her. No matter how many times you hear about them or see comedy made of them in movies and sitcoms, you have to go through it with someone you love to really know it's not a laughing matter. It seemed like pure torture. Even on the coldest nights we would find ourselves on the opposite spectrum of body temperature. I would be wearing warm clothing and still feeling a chill. Meanwhile, Lisa would be sitting in her nightgown, her face glistening with beads of sweat while moaning, "Feel me, I'm drenched!" Moments later, she'd be under the covers saying, "It's so cold." Throughout the night, her side of the covers would flop on and off repeatedly, while I would be comfortably tucked in.

Once, at two in the morning, she rolled over and exclaimed in frustration, "God, I'm shvitzing!" Now, I'm not Jewish, but I've picked up a few Yiddish words being married to her. In this situation, "shvitzing" would be translated to mean, "I wish these darn hot flashes would give me a break! They're making my life miserable!" That's a loose translation, of course.

I kissed her on her forehead, for I knew that as difficult as it was for me to deal with, menopause was a hundred times more difficult for her to live with. It caused me to remember something I agreed to sixteen years ago,". . . *for richer or poorer, in sickness or in health, till death do we part."* And even though this was not a sickness but a normal phase of life, I knew she was going to need me now more than ever.

Through the darkness, I saw her beautiful eyes filling with glistening tears. I said to her softly, "What's eight years? We can do that time standing on our heads."

Lawrence D. Elliott

True Love

Life is all about finding the right pill.

Shayla Johnson

I was forty-nine years old and in the throes of menopause when I first met Ed. We were sitting outside when he spotted a woman wearing a T-shirt that said, "I'm out of estrogen and I have a gun." He laughed. I said, "That's not funny." The expression on his face reflected confusion and fear. I explained to him that without my estrogen I could go a little crazy. Thankfully, Ed didn't jump up and run away.

I was on a monthlong vacation when this wonderful man entered my life. So when he asked me to stay two additional weeks, I happily agreed. Until, to my chagrin, I realized I had packed estrogen patches for only thirty days. Our host town was very small and had only one pharmacy. I immediately called my doctor and requested he send a new prescription.

The next day Ed and I went to pick up my much-needed hormone. I explained to Tom, the pharmacist, that I was from out of town and my doctor had called in the prescription. He went to his computer, typed in my name, then said, "I have no record of this."

I thought, *Oh my God, what am I going to do?* I worried unnecessarily, but it became immediately apparent that Ed's fear was greater than mine. I had the luxury of standing back as Ed leaned over the counter and very calmly but firmly told Tom, "You've got to find this prescription; we can't leave here without it!"

Tom realized this was a serious situation. He said, "Okay, let me check." After a few moments he said, "Wait. I do remember seeing this order. I didn't recognize the name and threw it away." Ed flew behind the counter and started rummaging through the trash basket, papers flying.

Finally, Ed said triumphantly, "I found it!" He handed the valuable document to Tom, pleading, "How soon can you fill this?"

"Two minutes," said Tom.

Knowing a calamity had been avoided, all three of us took a deep sigh of relief. At that time Ed had no idea what the ramifications of menopause were, but he was smart enough to know he didn't want to find out. We've been together ever since.

Unfortunately, hormone therapy does not cure all of the menopausal side effects. Poor Ed still finds it baffling when I go from crying tears of joy to tears of unhappiness in a split second, and absolutely nothing has happened to provoke either reaction. I explain through sobs and tears rolling down my face that I am fine. While my goal is to assure him I'm okay, I just confuse him more. Over time he's learned to wait patiently, knowing this emotional state will subside as quickly as it arrived.

Many times, I look in the mirror and still recognize the reflection, but have no idea who I am. One moment I'm a calm, sane, loving woman; the next, I'm wound as tight as a rubber band, ready to snap. I scream at everyone within earshot for no apparent reason. This is also frustrating for Ed; he isn't sure if he is living with Mother Teresa or Joan Crawford in "Mommie Dearest" mode.

I live in a constant state of confusion, not sure if I'm coming or going. My memory has taken a leave of absence. Being so forgetful, I've been given an exercise program, whether I want one or not. I walk upstairs, then can't remember why. I think hard to recall my purpose with no success. I give up and head back down the steps. Just as I reach the last step, I remember my original goal. I don't want to go back up the stairs, but if I don't do it now, I'll forget again. This aspect of menopause gives Ed an opportunity to tease me by saying, "Now are you ready to buy a one-story house?" He's no doubt earned the right to poke fun at me. For Ed, it was a positive menopause side effect, when, out of exhaustion, I finally agreed to move.

It's impossible to discuss menopause without mentioning hot flashes; Ed fears some night I will spontaneously combust and has taken out extra life insurance on me just in case. In addition, he is in search of flame-retardant bed linens to ensure he too doesn't become a casualty of menopause.

Fortunately, we both have maintained the most important ingredient for enduring menopause—a sense of humor. I'm very blessed to have such an understanding man in my life. Seven years after the drugstore scare, he still marks his calendar to make sure I refill my hormone prescription, not only because he loves me, but for his own self-preservation as well.

Tena Beth Thompson

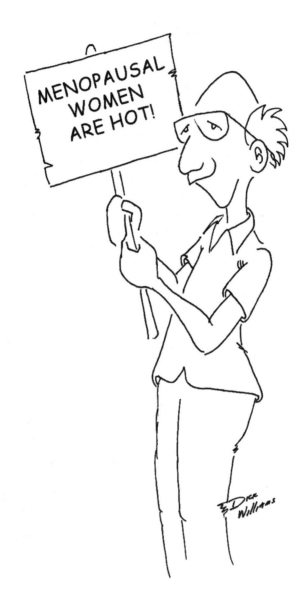

Raging Hormones, Raging Tears!

An archaeologist is the best husband any woman can have: the older she gets, the more interested he is in her.

Agatha Christie

So, okay, I've never been a beauty, nor have I acquired fame or fortune. Still, in the back of my mind was always the thought that any or all of these were possible if I wanted them badly enough. And I had plenty of time. That was until I looked into the mirror last week and saw someone else looking back at me. *Whose body was that anyway?* I said to myself.

At age fifteen, I promised myself I'd never be fat, so the lady in the mirror could not possibly be me. She had two chins and cheeks that could hold a melon in each. The eyes used to be vivid green but were now faded, and the color was not quite discernable. *How and when did all this happen? Why am I only now seeing it?* I started to cry. Two hours later I was still crying when my husband, James, came home for lunch.

In a concerned and slightly worried voice he asked,

"Honey, what's wrong? Why are you crying?"

I cried harder as I tried to speak and couldn't. Finally, I managed to blurt out, "I don't know. I just can't stop." The tears came faster and the sobs were more pathetic and louder than before.

James stood there looking helpless for a moment, then he came to me and attempted to give me a hug. I stepped back to avoid his reach as I spoke brokenly, "No, I don't deserve . . . *sob, sob* . . . a hug. How could you even . . . *sob* . . . bare to look at me, much less hug me? I'm so fat . . . *sob* . . . ugly . . . and . . . *sob* . . . and . . . *sob* . . . OLD!" I then covered my face with my hands, ran into the bathroom, and locked the door.

I could hear my husband in the kitchen preparing his own lunch as I continued to cry. Twice he came to the door to check on me. "Chris, I love you and neither of us are spring chickens, you know. We've been married for thirty-six years. You've given birth to three children. You've earned your pounds and wrinkles, and I love them all. Come on now and cheer up. You have a lot to be happy about," he said.

I bellowed, "Go away! I just want to cry!" I let out a few gut-wrenching wails for good measure.

I heard James hesitate, then he spoke softly through the closed door and through my torrential downpour of tears. "I'm leaving now, but remember that I love you and things will look different tomorrow. I'll call and check on you in a while. Are you sure there's nothing I can do to make you feel better?"

Now I was angry. Don't ask me why I was angry when James was being so sweet. I didn't know why—I just was! "Not unless you want to exchange bodies with me," I said. "And believe me, you wouldn't dare. *You* don't have to go through all of these horrid and dehumanizing changes. *You* are a *man*! *You* couldn't understand in a million years how I feel. Just go and let me cry!"

James replied, "I love you, and cry all you want, but you'll still be a woman and I'll still be a man—your man, the one you chose to spend your life with—for better or for worse."

He walked away mumbling something to himself about hormones and life's biggest challenge. I looked at my red splotchy face and my puffy, swollen eyes and detested what I saw reflected in the mirror even more than before. "I hate you. Who are you, anyway? I can't be this person!" I yelled at the mirror. And so it went for the better part of the day.

The phone rang several times, but I didn't even look at the caller ID screen to see who was calling. My head had begun to pound, and my nose was so stuffy I could barely breathe. I crawled into a little ball on the sofa and cried some more. The phone continued to ring. Finally, in exasperation, I picked it up and bellowed, "Hello?"

The caller said, "Sorry, wrong number," and hung up.

I held the receiver in my hand as I examined in my mind the sound of that familiar voice. *Sorry, wrong number?* I then realized it was James.

I began to laugh. Why it struck me as funny is anyone's guess. But I laughed and laughed until I was exhausted.

After reflecting upon my thirty-six years of marriage and the ups and downs James and I have experienced together, I felt my heart swell with love and admiration for this man. He was utterly unshakeable and so dependable—and he loved me.

Picking up the phone, I dialed my husband's cell phone number. "Hello, this is James," he answered.

In my softest and most loving voice, I said into the receiver, "I, Christine, take thee James to be my lawfully wedded husband. For richer, for poorer, in sickness and in health, for better and for worse, 'til . . ."

His strong voice interrupted, ". . . in hormones and

changes, till death do us part. I love you, Chris. Put on your sexiest nightshirt. I'm on my way home."

I heard the click, and my heart was so full of love, appreciation, and yes, acceptance. I'm not the same girl he married, that was a fact. But I am the same person, and he still loves me.

"Oh God, what I wouldn't give to have that black sexy nightgown I wore on our anniversary trip a few years ago," I mumbled, as I pulled two nightshirts from my drawer. I pondered my choices. One nightshirt depicted a housewife wearing a robe, slippers, and curlers in her hair. She held an empty cup in her hand, and the words read: "Just pour the coffee and back away slowly!" The kids had given me this one for Mother's Day. They all know I'm not a morning person.

The other nightshirt depicted a husband and wife in bed with the alarm clock blaring, but the wife is leaning toward the husband with a smile. The shirt reads, "Go ahead . . . make me late for work." *Which one will it be?*

Glancing at the clock, I decided there was time for me to rush to the department store two blocks away before James could get home. As I recalled, they had a great selection of lingerie. *Maybe something in black?* I grabbed my purse and keys as I hurried out the door. Before backing the car from the garage I caught a glimpse of myself in the rearview mirror—swollen eyes, a blotchy face, but a grateful heart. Giggling at the absurdity of it all, I wondered, *Do they even make sexy black nighties in extra large?*

Christine M. Smith

6

A SECOND
HELPING OF
MENTAL-PAUSE

Nobody ever died of laughter.

Max Beerbohm

Burn Baby Burn

If I have a thousand ideas and only one turns out to be good, I am satisfied.

Alfred Nobel

I missed the sexual revolution and the Age of Aquarius by about a decade, but I've made up for it by doing everything else too early. Now, at the age of forty-something, I found myself launched into an odd form of time warp; my daughters think me old, but I feel too young to be "middle-aged," whatever that is.

Sometime just after fire was invented and before Kotex had wings, and long before my cousin and I received "the talk," the two of us discovered my mother's box of tampons under the bathroom sink. When we inquired as to their use, my auntie and mother informed us that they were firecrackers. "Put those things back where you found them!" Big mistake telling two kids something was off-limits; try as we may, we just couldn't light these strange little firecrackers. But we did manage to ignite a large, but easily contained, brush fire in the backyard.

The years passed, as they tend to do. I graduated early

and started college at sixteen years of age, married at eighteen, and conceived my children early. Also at a young age, I had an aggressive and chronic case of endometriosis. I endured two laparoscopic surgeries, which were unsuccessful attempts to burn off the diseased tissue. After my third child was born, I was given two choices: 1) lifelong pain and possibly chemotherapy, or 2) a hysterectomy. I chose the latter, as it seemed less messy and painful in the long run. Besides, I rather liked my hair.

When I inquired about keeping my removed uterus and ovaries so I could give them a proper funeral, my gynecologist laughed, then he recited numerous regulations concerning the proper disposal of bio-hazardous materials. *Great,* I thought. *My womb was hazardous material!* I wondered what he would have called my meatloaf, but that's another cremation story. Still, I felt that losing my uterus and ovaries was the death of an era, and I wanted to properly mourn their passage. It took only a few weeks to recuperate from the surgery, but the feeling that I needed a ceremony of sorts to say goodbye to a part of me did not fade as quickly as the incision.

Now to tell this story correctly, it must be noted that our family has a large campfire pit in the backyard. We regularly roast hot dogs and marshmallows around the fire and occasionally light off a round or two of fireworks.

In a postmenopausal hot flash, I thought back to my childhood, then I glanced over at the fire pit. I knew what I had to do to memorialize my hysterectomy—I would have a party for my remaining boxes of feminine protection, a private, invitation-only wake for my little pals that had outlived their usefulness. Yeah, I could have given them to my friends, but there are just some things you don't give as leftovers, namely my meatloaf or a half-used box of panty liners!

You just gotta love my husband—he's such an overgrown Boy Scout. Realizing this was a special occasion, he built the perfect stack of kindling over the center of the pit, then tossed on a few logs, finally dousing it all with lots of lighter fluid. I then threw in all of my feminine paper products. Acting a touch odd, my husband was seemingly over-excited to fire her up! But I made him wait, as I needed to set the mood, and did so with "Disco Inferno," which blasted out of my tape deck (yes, I said tape deck—not CD player, not record player—give me a break).

Alas, the stage was set. We took our seats around the pit.

I lit the honorary match and tossed it in.

Whoosh!

Lord have mercy and ear plugs! Surprised, I stood straight up and had a sudden overwhelming need to cover my heart. I heard a twenty-one gun salute!

No . . . more like a hundred-and-one . . .

No, make that a small string of five hundred firecrackers, three bottle rockets, and one small roman candle. It suddenly dawned on me *that's* where my big Boy Scout had stashed the Fourth of July goodies. He was all smiles by my shocked reaction.

Things were exciting enough until the neighborhood dogs started barking and howling. Our kindly neighbor man sprinted right over (imagine Mr. Rogers wearing a pair of Nikes and baggy sweats, and you've got a visual on him) to see what the trouble was about, just in time to witness a winged panty liner launched into a blaze of glory. It landed right at his feet.

Lava-red with the sheer embarrassment of my spectacular ceremony, all I could manage to say to him as I exhaled and tried not to laugh was, "Gee, I guess they really do fly."

Although I never got to attend a Dead concert or burn my bra, I thoroughly enjoy the flashbacks of my life, and it's been cool, man, it's been really cool.

Jacqueline Michels

Wanted: One Inner Crone

Having stumbled my way into menstruation at the tender age of eleven, I had hoped to march into an early menopause. I figured twenty-five, thirty years tops, from start to finish. No such luck.

After almost forty years of checking the calendar on a monthly basis, I've had it. I'm more than ready to cast off the moon goddess and her cyclical visitations of fertility and embrace my inner crone.

Instead of obsessing about mundane things like lipstick shades, the numbers on the bathroom scale, and what to make for dinner, I will be transformed into a wise and caring earth goddess. I will shower the world with love and understanding. I will be one with nature. Not having to deal with monthly bloating and cravings would also be nice.

Unfortunately, my recalcitrant crone is not ready to embrace me back.

A few times over the last two years, she's danced into my life, only to glide out again three months later, leaving me once more to reach into the medicine cabinet for a tampon and circle another date on the calendar. I remain stranded in the purgatory of perimenopause, while my friends continue their journey into wisdom without me.

I've read dozens of books on menopause. I've increased my intake of soy to make the transition easier. I've even allowed the gray hairs to inch—okay, gallop—their way forward. What more does my tardy crone want?

In the meantime, she teases me with symptoms. Hot flashes ripple through my body and leave me breathless and sweating, with no gorgeous hunk in sight.

Lust I could handle. A malfunctioning internal thermometer renders me ridiculous, a radiator with no off button. I stand in front of the open refrigerator, waiting for its cooling breeze to return my body to some sense of normalcy, as I idly nibble on whatever leftovers have not evolved into new life forms.

Mood swings make getting up in the morning an adventure. I never know which one of me will climb out of bed—the good twin or the evil twin. My family and long-time friends point out that my middle name was always "moody," but I think they're just jealous that I have a built-in excuse for being miserable.

As a career cynic, I'm embarrassed to find myself crying at corny commercials or maudlin Hallmark cards. My prankster crone taunts me with meno "pauses," irritating lapses in memory that strike without rhyme or reason. I walk out of a room intent on retrieving an item, and a minute later I am reduced to wondering what I wanted. I prowl around the house, hoping the sight of something will trigger my memory. It doesn't.

Desperate, I bought a book on how to improve my memory, but my crafty crone descended long enough to hide the book. It's probably next to my missing ginkgo biloba pills, billed as an ancient Chinese memory enhancer—but only if I can find them.

Even if I could remember what I wanted, I probably couldn't find the right word for it. Yes, I am slowly losing my nouns, stolen, no doubt, by my tight-lipped crone. I am reduced to describing common objects as thingama-jigs or whatchamacallits or doohickeys. Pointing to objects in my own house is frustrating, but when I have to do it at work, it's humiliating.

UGH! I'm an English as a Second Language teacher and freelance writer. Words were my specialty. Now they're my nemesis. Luckily, my students are used to fumbling for words in English, and they sit patiently while I struggle to dredge up the right expression. And several other teachers are in the same thingamajig I'm in. That doohickey that floats on water, what is it?—boat!—they're in the same boat I'm in. So they nod sympathetically when I flounder.

Editors aren't quite as understanding. I find myself writing articles and putting Xs in places where I can't think of the term I want. Soon the Xs will outnumber the words.

As I sit on the couch, sobbing over some stupid made-for-TV movie, a chocolate bar in one hand and a XXXXXXX (to be filled in later, I hope) in the other, I wonder what else I can do to entice my treacherous crone. Buy a nicer couch? Eat imported chocolate? Install a satellite dish so I can watch better movies?

If my inner crone doesn't show up soon and turn me into a wise, compassionate, and loving woman, I'm going to wring her wrinkled little neck.

Harriet Cooper

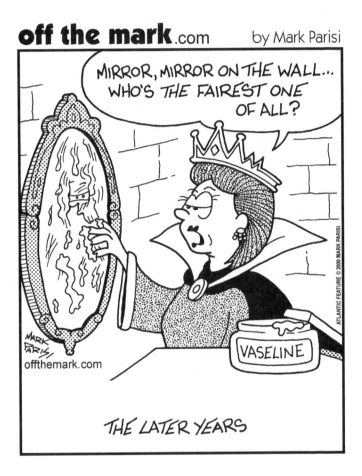

Snow-Capped Estrogen

When you get to the end of your rope, tie a knot and hang on.

Franklin D. Roosevelt

As many parents do each and every day, I was driving to my daughter's high school to pick her up. Parking and waiting for my teenager for those few quiet moments was going to be a welcome relief from my busy, dizzy life of being a single mother.

The going was slow because huge flakes of snow, unlike any I'd ever seen before, were falling. They were actually quite beautiful. It was a really great kind of snow to build snowmen because it was wet and held together really well.

As I entered the school parking lot, the wet snow reminded me of several days earlier, when my thirty-year-old son and I were outside my home. I was building a snow angel under the big purple plum tree while he was shoveling the driveway for me.

It was a very precious moment between a mother and her adult son. The air was absolutely still. You could have caught your breath in your hand and held it. The snow crunched happily under our feet. And, strangely, I felt very warm. While my son was seriously working in silence, I felt like a little girl under that beautiful old tree admiring my gorgeous snow angel. From behind me, I heard my son calmly ask, "Mom?"

I turned to see him smiling at me—and throwing a big snowball at the snow-laden tree branches above me! As you can well guess I was buried in snow! While digging my way out, I could hear my son's beautiful laughter. The driveway chore ended in a boisterous snowball fight!

Just as I shut my engine off, I was brought back to reality by a loud knock on my car window that startled me into bouncing my head off of the roof. The woman pounding on my window was clearly agitated about something. I rolled down my window, and she immediately asked if I had a cell phone. I didn't and asked her what was wrong. She quickly explained that a man had rear-ended her car at the corner traffic light and had followed her into the parking lot to exchange information, but that he was clearly high on either alcohol or drugs.

Well, that got me going. Imagine, driving in a school zone under the influence at three o'clock in the afternoon! I immediately got out of my car, fuming. I told her to go look for a cell phone and call 911, or ask one of the teenagers to alert school staff.

I approached the man's vehicle and knocked on his window. His car was still running. He rolled his window down, and I asked him if he had had anything to drink. He said that he hadn't. His eyes were bright red. I asked him again if he had been drinking, and he admitted that he had. He said that he was visiting from out of town and had just left an all-night party and was "just tired." Meanwhile, his breath almost knocked my socks off!

I was so infuriated that he might have hurt someone. "Sir (I was a regular "Cops" viewer and used the phrases I thought was suitable), I want you to turn off your car and give me your keys," I ordered.

He looked at me and sneered, "You can't tell me what to do!"

I repeated, "Turn off your car and give me the keys!" This time I added more authority to my voice. He was not going to shut his car off or give me the keys. *Where on earth was the woman who went to call the police?* I thought. I walked out to the entrance of the parking lot and stopped the first vehicle driving toward me. I asked the two men in the truck to block the entrance until the police came. They agreed.

I trekked back to the car through the heavy snow that was continuing to fall. Irritated, I again demanded that he give me his keys. I was envisioning some innocent teenager, maybe mine, being hit by this man. I blew!

"Who do you think you are asking me for my keys?" he slurred.

I reached through the open window and grabbed his keys from the ignition before he knew what hit him. "I am a mother," I proclaimed, "and I am in full-throttle menopause. I am making a citizen's arrest. Stay right where you are, buddy!"

He sat quietly until the police arrived and statements were filed. Afterward, I got in my car and headed home with my beautiful daughter. About one mile from the school, still thinking about what I had done, I started to shake. I yelled out, "What was I thinking?!"

"Mom, you did real good back there," Danielle said. "I'm proud of you, except . . ."

"Except what, honey?" I asked.

She hesitated a moment. "Well, you did great, except you have about a foot of snow piled on top of your hat!"

I began to laugh. I don't know how anyone could have taken me seriously looking the way I did. It must have been my estrogen look.

Glady Martin

I'm Not Going

The door of change is open,
But I choose not to go.
It's just too soon to think about.
I'm not that old, you know.

I'll not march forth toward menopause,
That malicious badge of aging.
I won't step 'cross that threshold
Into hormones that are raging.

I can't give in, I must resist,
Must turn my back and flee.
I must find another route and
Avoid maturity.

I'll dye my hair a rich dark hue.
I'll paint my nails bright pink.
I'll wear the latest fashion trends,
And pierce my nose, I think.

I'll eat more fruits and vegetables
And diet to size ten.

My innards will not have a clue
That changes should begin.

The door of change will surely close
If I appear quite young.
If in doubt I'll get tattooed
And wear diamonds in my tongue.

No, I shall not go right now
Through the door beyond my youth.
I'll stay right here another year
And deny genetic truth.

Why is it so hot in here?

Rachel S. Neal

Menopausal Moments

It was the best of times, it was the worst of times.

Charles Dickens

After suffering through several years of pain, not to mention inconvenience, I finally decided to take my doctor's advice and have elective surgery to correct one of those notorious female problems. Several weeks before the procedure, my doctor gave a detailed accounting of what the surgery involved, what I could expect in terms of recovery, and what preoperative measures I would be required to undergo. I listened intently but asked few questions. So, when my physician began describing the injection that I would receive the next day, an injection that would put my body in a menopausal state for several weeks, I simply nodded my head as if I were completely aware of what a menopausal state might involve. Hot flashes, night sweats, and mood swings for a few weeks were nothing compared to what I had been experiencing for years. I quickly discovered how very wrong I was.

For several days after receiving the injection, I noticed absolutely no change in my physical or emotional state. We were a normal, happy family. I even bragged to my husband that I was going to have it made when I really did enter that phase of my life. Based on this experience, I would almost certainly be one of those few women who never even realized that they were experiencing "the change."

Life proceeded merrily along. Then the inevitable happened. I awoke in the middle of the night from a deep sleep. My pajamas were soaked. I felt an intense heat that I had never before felt. It seemed to be coming from somewhere deep inside my body and was rapidly spreading to my extremities. I panicked. *I hadn't had the surgery yet, so this couldn't be attributed to post-surgery infection,* I thought. *I must have contracted some horrible bacterial illness whose symptoms include a high fever!* Knowing that death was obviously imminent, I writhed and moaned, kicking off covers and sheets.

Then I noticed that my husband was still asleep. He was resting comfortably while his wife, whom he had promised to love and cherish in sickness, lay next to him dying. *Could he not sense that I was in a near-death condition? How dare he lie there snoring while I was feverish and in need of immediate medical attention!* Just as I was rearing back to kick him out of bed to attend to his ailing wife, it suddenly hit me. *I'm having a hot flash! This is a night sweat!* For a few brief seconds, I still contemplated waking my husband using a slightly less violent method. After all, he was surely somehow at fault for my misery. But, as the heat subsided degree by degree, my sanity returned at slow intervals. *So this was what my mother had been experiencing.* Suddenly, I understood what she had been going through. Tears filled my eyes as I recalled my own lack of sympathy toward her complaints in recent months. I sniffled and snorted, now in need of a tissue but too drained to move. An involuntary leg spasm of some sort, however, resulted in contact with my slumbering husband's body. He awakened and attended to all my needs, as he most certainly should have.

Over the next few weeks, I had the opportunity to have a full-fledged menopausal experience. When I was not crying about failing to eat the yogurt before the expiration date or bawling because I had bought purple grape juice rather than the white variety, I alternated between periods of euphoria and deep, dark depression. I had many sleepless nights, and my poor husband may have accidentally gotten pushed out of bed a couple of times to bring me tall glasses of ice water and cool clothes. My children, who happen to be very perceptive, learned quickly to watch my face for sudden changes in color and expression. They knew when to avoid me, which, unfortunately, was frequently, and they became very close to the neighbors that summer. The dog and I simply renewed our relationship after the effects of the injection wore off weeks later.

The surgery and my brief introduction to menopause were ultimately worth the interruption to my otherwise normal life. My female problems were corrected, and I now have a profound respect for any woman who is going through menopause, as does my husband. I am not, however, looking forward to that phase of my life when nature, rather than medical science, says that it is time, a time that is approaching more rapidly than I care to think about. At least my family will be better prepared. My children will be old enough to move out and not be dependent on neighbors for refuge. My husband will have time to buy a comfortable couch on which to sleep uninterrupted, and, as for the dog, there is still a little time to work that out!

Terri Duncan

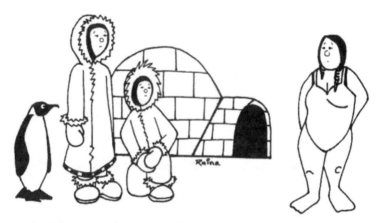

"Your mother must be having another one
of those 'Hot Flash Things.'"

To Err Is Human

It's only when the tide goes out that you learn who's been swimming naked.

Warren Buffett

Menopause was giving me grief, but I was managing okay, or so I thought.

One October evening, the main dish I was going to prepare for dinner was lentils with chunky bits of ham simmered to perfection. Lentils were one of my hubby, Ed's, favorite childhood foods. I was excited about surprising him with the dish.

Stews, roasts, and soups always came out perfect when they were cooked in my stainless steel oven. I retrieved the old Dutch oven, the one my grandma had made so many of her famous homemade meals in during my own childhood. Once my perfectly square bites of ham were placed in the old pot, I filled the antique with the precise amount of water and spices. I then went to the cupboard for the lentils that I had neatly stored in a Ziploc bag. This was actually our second meal of the delicious beans; however, it had been so long ago since I'd prepared them, I'd nearly forgotten how to cook them. I opened the unmarked Ziploc and gently poured the beans into the mixture.

Before long, I began to smell the aroma of the ham. It smelled good. Even the dog seemed enchanted by the wonderful fragrance.

My teenage son soon came through the front door. "Mom, what are you cooking for dinner?" he asked in a displeased tone.

"I'm fixing lentils," I said, with an upbeat attitude. "Ed's grandmother used to make them."

"They stink," he said, wrinkling his nose in disgust as he left the room.

Removing the lid from my old pot, I inhaled deeply. Instantly, my stomach turned. *What the heck?* I asked myself. *They smelled okay a minute ago.*

I remembered that the last time I had fixed Ed's child-hood favorite, they had tasted pretty good. I shrugged my shoulders, replaced the lid, and waited to hear my husband's car pulled into the driveway.

I didn't have to wait long. Ed walked through the door and quickly found the pot. He lifted the lid. "What are you making?"

"Lentils! Can't you tell?"

"Oh," he said returning the pot's cover. "The beans were on the bottom. I couldn't see them," he said, never asking about the stench that hung in the air.

An hour later, my son came out of his bedroom and sat next to Ed and me on the couch. By then, the stink in the house was overwhelming "I don't want to eat anything that smells like that," he said.

"They're good." I assured him. "Ed loves them. His grandma used to write his initials in ketchup on them when he was a little boy."

"They smell like burnt peanuts! I'm outta here!"

"Where are you going?"

"I'm going to get something to eat. I can't eat that stuff."

Quickly, I ran to the kitchen to see if the lentils were burning. Stirring the pot, I noticed that although my supper wasn't burnt, the beans were still as hard as they were when I began cooking them. I returned the lid and joined my husband on the sofa. My stomach was beginning to growl with hunger.

"Are they done yet?" Ed asked. "They've been cooking for over two hours."

"Soon," I answered, wondering if my prediction would be true. Allowing another thirty minutes to pass, I asked my husband to check on dinner.

"I'm not sure, honey. They're still kind of hard," he said after careful examination. Knowing full well the tiny beans should be nothing but mush at this point, I asked him to taste them.

"Barb," I heard him say, "these aren't lentils."

"They are too."

"No they aren't!"

"Well, what are they then?" I demanded as I walked into the kitchen.

"I have no idea, but they aren't lentils."

"Let me see," I said, grabbing the spoon from my husband. I lifted the rock-like beans from the bottom of the pot. He was right. Whatever it was that had been stinking the house to high heaven was not lentils.

I opened the cupboard. I was positive I'd only cooked half of the little round beans the last time I'd fixed them. *They couldn't have spoiled; beans last for a long time,* I reassured myself. *Ziplocs are airtight.* I moved the items around in the cupboard. Suddenly, I spotted the flavored croutons that I had used in the delicious salad I'd made a week or so earlier, and then the empty spot next to them. In an instant, I knew where I'd failed. I hung my head and turned to Ed.

"I know what they are," I said in a meek voice. "We'd better go out for supper."

"What are they?"

"Sunflower seeds!" I answered, shaking my head in disbelief that I had managed such an idiotic mistake.

Ed laughed. "How in the world?"

"Menopause," I said as I grabbed my coat. Without muttering another word, my smart, wonderful husband followed me out the door.

Adding insult to injury, later that evening upon retiring to our bedroom, Ed rubbed his stomach. "I've got heartburn," he said, not sounding too well.

Great, I thought. *Probably from digesting those sunflower seeds.* Again, being the sweet wife that I am, I offered to get him some Maalox tablets. I tossed the bottle to him.

"Do I take one or two?"

"Two," I answered.

Doing as he was told, Ed opened the bottle and popped the tablets into his mouth. As he chewed, a terrible look came over his face. "Are you sure you're supposed to chew these things?"

"Of course I'm sure; they're antacids."

"They don't taste very good," he murmured between bites, the look on his face getting worse.

"Let me see the bottle," I said, taking it from him. I started to laugh.

Ed sat up instantly. "What? What's so funny?"

I couldn't stop laughing. I had tossed him my bottle of Women's One-A-Day vitamins!

Barbara Wenger

Keep the Change

There once was a woman
with worries galore,
who went to her doctor
as if at death's door.

"Now tell me your symptoms,"
the doctor replied.
And here's what she said
as she trembled and cried:

"Early one morning,
I went number one,
and I heard some clinking,
and when I was done,

"I looked in the toilet,
and guess what I saw. . .
a small pile of pennies,
and I was in awe!

"And then the next morning,
I heard the same sound,

and there in the toilet,
some nickels I found!

"And on the third morning,
I saw a few dimes,
and after that quarters
a number of times!"

"There's no need to worry,"
said old Doctor Bliss.
"A woman your age
will experience this.

"It's really quite normal.
I know that it's true.
There's no need to fear
what has happened to you.

"See, you're nearly fifty,
and this isn't strange.
To put it quite simply,
you've gone through the change."

Albert Van Hoogmoed

Poor Clyde

It was finally Friday afternoon. It had been a very long week at the manufacturing company where I was employed as the purchasing manager.

One of my responsibilities was to address all the correspondence to and from our vendors. We had been having problems getting product out of one of our sole-source suppliers. The boss asked me to write a letter and tactfully remind them that they were not performing to our agreement, and also that we needed components for our production line as soon as possible.

I found it quite difficult to write a tactful letter. I wanted to scream at them, but of course, that couldn't happen. I was tired and irritable. I had not slept well the entire hectic week, as night sweats were robbing me of much-needed rest. I seemed to have one decent week a month. But lately, my emotional levels could hit manic highs and rock-bottom lows in one fifteen-minute span, which was unusual for me. This whole menopausal thing was becoming very troublesome. They didn't even call it menopause yet; it was *perimenopause,* as if *that* made a difference. I had tried different medications to find relief, but the doctor could not find the right combination. My doctor thought herself humorous, teasing, "What's the matter, Bonnie? Are you losing all your friends?"

Very funny, I thought, in my cranky state of mind. The only people who understood me were the ones in the same midlife dilemma. Some friends and I joked about staying away from each other for five years in order to retain our friendships until this crisis passed. This is when it's a blessing to have friends in all age groups.

Anyway, I had to get this letter written before I could go home—and I was ready for the weekend. Typing intently, I tried to use just the right words with the right amount of firmness, but not be negative in tone.

Concentrating hard, I felt a presence behind me but ignored it since I wanted to finish the last sentence. *BAMM!* The loud bang of a hammer hitting my desk sent me straight up out of my chair. Instantly furious, and without as much as a second of hesitation, I clenched my fist, whirled around and punched the unsuspecting maintenance man in the stomach with every bit of strength in me. I hadn't even thought but simply reacted in a moment of anger. If it had been the company owner, I would have been in a great deal of trouble as he was a small man and not in the best physical shape. Luckily it turned out to be Clyde, a very fit fellow who rode motorcycles on the weekends. Even at that, he made a loud "Oof" and bounced back a couple of feet when I landed the punch. We just looked at each other; I was flabbergasted at what I had just done, and Clyde looked at me with total disbelief. Neither of us spoke, but I could feel the color rising in my face as I realized what had just taken place. I felt foolish, but deep down, still a *tiny bit* justified.

"I'm very sorry," Clyde said slowly. "I must have really scared you."

"Yes, you did," I answered with a sheepish smile. "I'm sorry." Trying to recover some professionalism, I asked,

"Was there something you needed from me?"

"You know what, I think it can wait until Monday," he said.

Trying to make light of a totally embarrassing situation, I said, "Thanks, Clyde, I would appreciate that. Please be more careful next time. I don't like to be surprised."

Well, time passed, and the doctor did find the right hormone prescription to settle my nerves and allow me to rest better. Two fibroid tumors were removed, which gave me relief from the pain I had been experiencing. Menopausal symptoms lessened to tolerable and eventually to minuscule. I even managed to keep most of my friends and family through the ordeal.

At work, Clyde and I remained amicable. He treated me with the utmost respect, but, much to my chagrin, he never let me forget the day I delivered him that sucker punch.

Bonnie Nester

Keeping Abreast of Change

"You're in perimenopause," my gynecologist told me at my annual checkup.

"But I feel so lousy! I'm tired and moody! And my brain cells seem to be in the midst of a mass exodus!"

"Don't worry," she reassured me. "That's normal. Perimenopause means preparing for menopause."

What kind of babble was that? Is periwinkle preparing for blue? Being informed that I was not yet experiencing menopause did not assuage my hot flashes, fuzzy memory, moodiness, fatigue, or occasional panic attacks.

"Let's speed this up," I said.

"You can't," she answered. "Your blood work confirms that you're just one of those lucky women who will not reach menopause until your mid-fifties."

WHAT? How could I be fifty-two with miles to go before reaching this new period (or lack of) in my life? My sister, who's three years younger, had already passed menopause with flying colors.

I wasn't pleased. My doctor advised, "Just let nature take its course. Eventually, your symptoms will become more noticeable, your periods erratic, but you'll muddle through." *Muddle through?* I was not happy.

Soon after, I was rushing to prepare for an early-morning business meeting. In between getting my kids up and dressed, feeding them breakfast, and walking my youngest to the bus stop, I was trying to determine which outfit camouflaged the most body flaws while still qualifying as "appropriate business attire." I opted for black pants, chunky black heels, and my favorite crème-colored silk blouse.

Once the kids were gone, I slipped out of my sweats, showered, and donned my slacks and black knee-high hose. Despite limited sleep (another perimenopausal perk) on this particular morning, I was at full speed by 7:30 AM, or so I thought, until I started to slip on a sports bra before remembering that I needed to wear a "real" bra!.

I needed to leave by 8:30 but still had to address my hair, makeup, and nails. I somehow had the presence of mind not to risk getting foundation on my blouse. I left it on the hanger and slipped into my short white mini-robe, tying the matching belt into a bow. I blow-dried my hair in front of the mirror and once it was dry, I placed it in a ponytail atop my head (à la Pebbles Flintstone) while I waited for my electric curlers (from 1976!) to heat up. What a sight!

The phone rang. My husband was out of town and needed help. A sample had accidentally been shipped to our home instead of to him. He asked if I could listen for the FedEx truck, due to arrive any minute, sign for the package, then get to the FedEx store and pay for an overnight delivery to his hotel. "No problem," I told him. We chatted briefly, wished each other a good day and hung up.

I returned to the mirror—my lower half dressed, my upper half protected by my mini-robe—when I realized I hadn't plucked my eyebrows in a very long time. *Funny, they didn't seem to need it,* I thought. My eyebrows, along with my lips, were getting thinner. I was happy to see that at least something on my body was going in that direction! I never enjoyed the sting from plucking my eyebrows and was happy I didn't need to pluck now (at last . . . a perimenopausal perk!).

Relief had just settled in when I first caught glimpse of . . . *it!* A thin, baby-fine piece of hair was stuck at an odd angle underneath my chin. I tried brushing it off. It remained. To my horror, I realized that it had, unbeknownst to me, taken up residence. *Eyebrows are thinning near the top of my head, but hair is now sprouting on my chin. How long has it been there? Am I the last person on the planet to notice it?*

"You're going DOWN, suckah!" I said, grabbing my magnifying mirror and tweezers. I tried to grasp it. What a sly little bugger! The clock was ticking. I finally managed to grasp the wispy thing and yanked it out. YOUCH! My eyes teared. The underside of my chin was completely red! I wondered if it would grow back . . . or worse, bring friends! Like I'd seen my husband do many times after shaving, I grabbed a small piece of Kleenex, ran it under cold water, and placed it on my sore chin, deciding to wait until the redness disappeared to apply my makeup. I hurriedly painted my nails. Just then, the doorbell rang.

FedEx! I'd forgotten! I raced from the bedroom to the other end of the house, shouting, "Be right there!"

When I reached the front door, I carefully, but swiftly, opened the door, quickly letting the doorknob go to protect my wet nails. As the door swung past me, the larger belt loop of my minirobe silently slid over the doorknob, and the belt untied. There I stood, in front of the delivery man and the world, in black pants, hose . . . and . . . *ta da* . . . my beige bra. I was so busy trying to protect my nails, sign the form, and grab the package, several seconds passed before reality hit.

"Uh . . ." the FedEx guy stammered.

I was mortified. As I reattached my robe, I tried to say, "Do you need my signature?" but somehow the words came out, "Would you like my autograph?" The poor man, probably thought I was a faded striptease artist craving attention. He stared at the floor as he shoved the clipboard into my hand. (Where are sinkholes when you need them?)

My only solace after my "morning outing" was that at least he didn't see my chin hair! (FedEx now delivers to our neighborhood in the late afternoon!)

Debra Simon

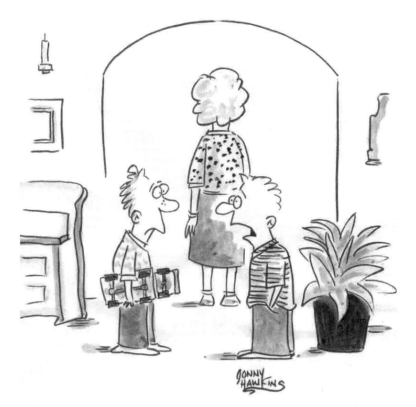

"When Aunt Martha kisses me it gives me a warm,
fuzzy feeling—mainly from the stubble on her chin."

Menopause Revenge

The secret of a happy marriage remains a secret.

Henny Youngman

About five years ago, before we had a yard service, my husband, Bob, and I worked in the yard every weekend. One weekend we would mow, the next we would weed-eat the edges and clean the flower beds—you know the drill.

I love flowers and have huge trees with flower beds around most of the yard. Bob was on the riding lawnmower mowing the front lawn (we live in the country so we have about an acre to keep). Since he was working so hard, I decided to get him a huge glass of ice tea. As I was heading to the front of the yard from the back door, I rounded the corner of the house and instantly knew something was wrong. It took me a couple of menopausal seconds to realize what my darling husband had done. Where there used to be two feet of flowers around the biggest tree in our front yard, there was nothing but little green blades sticking up. I knew immediately it was because he didn't want to get his rear end off the riding mower and use the push mower.

As I approached him, I could barely see because everything I saw was red. "What in the world did you do to my flower bed?" I asked him. His Aggie answer—are you ready for this—"I didn't mean to."

"Didn't mean to" means you mow a few flowers down and go, "Uh-oh!" You don't ride the mower around the whole darn tree until there are no more flowers. What a goober!

Needless to say, I didn't give him the ice tea, but returned to the house in a steaming rage. I knew I had to do something to aggravate him, something that would make me feel good just enough not to commit murder. *I could get a bat*, I thought. *No, he has to work. And if I cut up his easy chair, I'd just have to buy a new one, and people would find out just how crazy I really am.*

Then it hit me. About two weeks ago, Bob had spent hours putting little tools, washers, and everything else men use to build things into a tool box. The thing had to weigh at least 100 pounds. Everything was in its place, and he was so proud that he could find all of them. REVENGE!

I went to the front window and looked out at least six times while I dragged his huge tool box to the backyard. He was still mowing and acting like he had done nothing wrong. After I managed to drag the toolbox to the back yard, I picked out pieces of little tools in handfuls and threw them into the yard, you know, so the mower would sling them even farther and maybe break that riding mower he was still riding. After I finished throwing everything from each of the compartments, I turned the rest of the tool box over.

Finally, I had peace! I didn't have to commit any kind of murder or be committed. I felt so good that I went into the house and started dinner—*smug* comes to mind.

It was about thirty minutes later when this man, with a vein sticking out of the side of his neck, came into the house. I knew immediately this was not the time to say, "Na na na na boo boo." In so many words (use your imagination), he asked why I had thrown his tools out into the yard.

I very calmly said, "I didn't mean to."

Bob turned around and walked out of the room as though he had developed some sort of affliction that would not allow his legs to move. I know he had murder on his mind, but he knew he couldn't get away with it—I had already written a note, just in case.

To this day, not one of my flowers has been mowed down again. And it was a very long time before he would laugh about the episode. Every now and again, when I find a washer or a tool out in the yard, I'll hold it up and say, "Hey, Bob, is this yours?"

I am definitely menopausal, plus I'm a Texan. Both of them together can be pretty dangerous.

Connie Parish

7

WHO TURNED UP THE HEAT?

No river can return to its source, yet all rivers must have a beginning.

American Indian Proverb

To Fan or Not to Fan

Many a small thing has been made large by the right kind of advertising.

Mark Twain

It started again when my husband was in the living room watching television, his favorite pastime. That warm feeling was coming back, from head to toe. I thought, *Oh no, not again!*

The sweat rolled down my armpits, then my forehead. I went from warm to 1,000 degrees in seconds. It was so hot that I stripped off my soaked blouse just to try and cool down. That did little good, so I proceeded to take off the rest of my clothes. I frantically looked for the fan and realized it was in the living room, and so was my husband!

Up to this point I had been having a few episodes of hot flashes, but they hadn't been so bad that my husband had yet noticed. But this episode was a really bad one, and I just had to get to that fan. Frantic, I streaked into the living room, in between my husband and his beloved television, yelling "Hot! Hot!" I felt a sudden wave of cool relief as the fan sweep across my face and upper body—I was in hot-flash heaven. But when I turned around, to my surprise I found my husband standing in his undies! "What do you think you're doing?" I asked. "You yelled 'hot!' and I thought you wanted me to play fireman!" was his answer.

I know he was trying to be romantic, but I just started laughing. He looked puzzled. I then explained to him I was going through "the change." We went out that very day and bought a fan for every room in the house so there would never be another confused signal.

Husbands? Ya gotta love 'em!

Ginger Kenchel

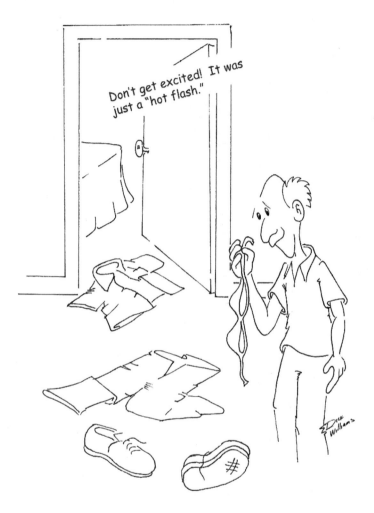

The Adventures of Swamp Woman

"I think I'll start wearing scuba gear to bed," my husband said the other night. "I don't want to drown."

"Ha, ha," I replied. But I could sympathize. I wish I could protect myself from myself. Hardly a night passes where I am not awakened awash in steamy sweat. I have turned into Swamp Woman, starring in the *Curse of the Crone*.

That would make a great title for a horror movie. Let's see . . . *Swamp Woman is a perfectly normal person until her mid-fifties when she suddenly straps on a backpack and goes trekking in Borneo. There she barely escapes being dragged out of a longboat by a rabid crocodile, but not before she is injected with the jungle virus through the crocodile's bite. Now, each night, she becomes an oozing creature of the jungle waters looking for relief. She turns first to her family for support, nearly drowning her husband in a hug when all she really wants to do is assure herself that she is still desirable. She slimes her way to her children's bedrooms, hoping to get the help she needs, but cannot find a single dry towel. In her mad, wet resolve, she vows to experiment until she discovers the herbs that will ease the heat raging inside her. She uses her friends as test subjects and leaves a trail of chemically altered mutants behind her. . . .*

I haven't figured out the ending yet, but just think of

the possibilities for special effects. We could leave out the part that menopause plays in this; it's much better fictionalized.

Menopause has brought out in me a whole host of skills that I never knew I possessed. Besides dreaming up screenplays, I am now a fashion consultant for my friends who are shifting into the "wet season." We choose clothes by how little they show the damp spots. Black is the preferred color. Twin sets are good because the outer sweater can be removed when the heat rises and then popped back on when the under sweater soaks through and the chills start. Beading is concealing on fancy wear and a shawl adds just the right fashion touch, especially when shoulders begin to dissolve atop a slinky evening gown.

I have also become a stress counselor for women's groups, offering understanding and techniques to those who are experiencing the transition into mature womanhood and need help coping. And my years of yoga have at last come in handy. "Breathe," I tell them. "Focus. Find your inner puddle . . . I mean . . . your core." These workshops have a de-stressing effect on me as well once I get going, but I must admit that planning for them makes me nervous enough to have flash attacks beforehand.

My mother never prepared me for this. Back then women didn't talk about such things. They endured in silence or threw tantrums but did not reveal the source of their distress. In all fairness, maybe my mother didn't have hot flashes. Not every woman does. Somewhere between 50 and 85 percent of women experience hot flashes and night sweats. That means a lucky 15 to 50 percent escape with their internal thermometer intact.

My daughter won't be able to say that about me. She has seen me turn scarlet over the salad course at a restaurant. She has watched her mother prance around in a T-shirt and shorts during a winter freeze when she, herself, was sitting in the kitchen wearing a hat and scarf. She knows what is going on. She reminds me to breathe. I think it is important to share the full life cycle. Let my daughter see how I deal with maturing. It will give her something to laugh about when she is in the same position, if she is, and maybe offer some insights into the joys and challenges that come with female aging.

And there are joys. Like knowing who you are, *at last.* Like having the freedom to explore parts of you that were kept in check by the responsibilities of youth and middle age. Appreciating the resonance of "long-time" friendships. Feeling the throb of life within the changes going on.

So, back to the adventures of Swamp Woman . . . *We last saw her experimenting in the laboratory looking for the precise combination of ingredients to halt the insidious, creeping night sweats. She has been reading about cooling substances from the annals of herbalism, Ayurveda, and traditional Chinese medicine. She brews a mixture of black cohosh, basil, coconut oil, dried peaches, and rose buds. She cools the bubbling mixture, then purees and strains it into a glass. It looks like toxic sludge, but to Swamp Woman it represents hope. Now for the test. Does she drink it or slather it all over her body? The fire is stoking itself inside her like an alien being. Do it. Do it now! She holds up the glass. It is time. . . .*

The tension is unbearable. I think I'll sit quietly and do my breathing practice. And while I'm calm, maybe I can come up with further adventures: *Flood and Fire in the Suburbs, The Revenge of Swamp Woman,* or perhaps, and this is my personal favorite, *Swamp Woman Out of Control.* Who knows where this could lead. Perhaps I'll have a whole new career. I believe in seeing things in a positive light. When life hands out lemons, I'll be the first in line at the lemonade stand. More ice, please.

Ferida Wolff

Hot Flashes and Promises

It is good to have an end to journey toward, but it is the journey that matters in the end.

Ursula K. LeGuin

I felt silly getting married at age fifty. *Weren't weddings for sweet young things with the rosy blush of youth still in their cheeks?* I thought. Those were the images I saw on the covers of wedding magazines, after all. Here I was getting married, with two kids old enough to start thinking about finding their own life partners. I had gray hair and wrinkles, for goodness sake. And yet, I wanted to celebrate finding that perfect love, a love that made me young again, even though my mirror tried to deny it.

We could have gone to the county courthouse and had it all over and done with in an hour, but I wanted to mark that day with a real wedding—nothing formal, but a wedding with at least some of the usual trappings. I wanted my friends and family with me. I wanted a cake and a reception. I wanted a "wedding-ish" dress. I even wanted little plastic swans, although I never did figure out what to do with them. But what I didn't want was to look ridiculous. *Could a fifty-year-old with flabby upper arms be a beautiful bride?*

The dress was the biggest ordeal. No, I didn't want a floor-length, lace-and-pearls bridal gown, but why did every salesperson immediately lead me to the "mother of the bride" section? *Did both the florist and caterer also assume that it was my daughter who was getting married?*

After finding a suitable dress, thanks to considerable guidance from my most fashion-conscious friend, the rest of the preparations fell easily into place. I addressed invitations and fussed over details, feeling at once both excited and unsure. *Was I being ridiculous?* My family and friends offered me nothing but support and even my kids seemed to approve. But my lingering insecurity had me comparing myself to the images of the beautiful, young brides I began to notice everywhere. I really didn't think I measured up.

The last-minute preparations were a whirlwind. My dear friend Marylou did my hair and makeup. My creative sister Janelle decorated the cake and took pictures. Mary made up beautiful centerpieces for the tables and a bridal bouquet with my favorite flowers. My other good friends helped the harried caterer finish setting the tables after his assistant failed to show up. With all the excitement, I forgot most of my insecurities. Even as I struggled into the spandex undergarment that was supposed to rein in my wayward fat, I was only thinking about how happy I was to be marrying the man of my dreams, surrounded by all these loving people.

It was a simple and beautiful outdoor wedding near the shores of Lake Tahoe. The weather was perfect. A late winter had delayed the wildflowers, which still bloomed profusely in early July. And once we had made it through the ceremony, with just a few forgotten lines, I was thrilled and relieved and so happy that we'd chosen a "real" wedding.

Everyone told me I looked beautiful, radiant, glowing. And I did feel beautiful and radiant, almost like . . . oh yes, a hot flash! With a knowing smile on my lips, I happily thanked one and all. There's more than one way to get the rosy blush of youth in your cheeks!

Marjorie Woodall

It's a Manopause Thing

Do all things with love.

Og Mandino

Spring comes to the island in interludes of fine weather
followed by bitter winds and rain, often several shifts of
each in an hour. It is our custom on the weekends to take
the dog and walk to an area called "Butler Main." Once a
logging road, it's now blocked off on either side to prevent
dumping, allowing the natural world to grow back. My
husband insists that I only walk there when he is with me,
isolated a track as it is. He says it's because of the bears,
but I know it's a man thing.

So one morning we dressed appropriately in layers.
White T-shirt, followed by a long-sleeved shirt followed by
a vest and jacket. The dog danced around as we also dug
out gloves and headbands, and with that and the walking
sticks, we were out the door. We were approaching the
road when it came—that growing flash of warmth. My
friend told me she thought they were more like hot surges
then flashes, and I had to agree. I didn't all of a sudden get
hot. I got hot in layers.

The gloves and headband were stuffed in my pocket as we surged ahead. The wind was whipping up the tree branches along the road. Great! Welcome the wind! By the time we reached the entrance I had undone my coat, and not long after that had it hung on my arm as it brushed away my sweat.

I chattered on as we walked, noting the coming of new plants and the bones from a deer dragged here long ago. The dog scurried after wild rabbits as I felt another wave approaching. I took off the last of my garments; I was down to my thin white T-shirt. The wind blew and felt *sooo* good I couldn't help but dance around in it. Suddenly I realized that my husband had been saying less and less. In fact one might say I was getting the silent treatment. I turned to see him standing there, scowling at me. In his hand were his jacket, vest, and outer shirt, and his skin was a frostbitten hue of pale blue accompanied by goose bumps.

"For goodness sake, put on your jacket!" he said to me. He stood with his teeth chattering. It was then that I understood. Not to look weak, he had adjusted his layers according to mine. It was a "manopause" thing.

"Dear," I said quietly, "it's not the weather, it's my menopause. I'm flashing now, and the wind is the only thing keeping me from spontaneously combusting. I'm sure it'll pass by the time we get to the end of the trail. Meanwhile, there's no one else around. Put your jacket back on. I won't tell."

Gratefully, he nodded and layered himself once more. By the end of the road, I, too, was finally feeling the cold. I put my clothes back on just as the rain began to fall, and we were again visible to other country dwellers.

Yes, spring does have its seasonal outbursts, but the fall of a woman's life can also be as changeable as a gusty, sunny day along the Butler Main.

Nancy Bennett

Déjà Vu

"Menopause is tough, right?"

When I'm asked that question, I'm not so sure. One day in 1973, I discovered I was pregnant. In my mid-twenties, it felt like the right time to start a family. My husband exhibited his pride by sticking out his chest, while my tummy began to pop a special bulge. Almost from day one, my olfactory senses revolted if they encountered the untoward smells of frying bacon or smokestack cigars. Oh, the horrid stench! Yuck!

Nausea and spinning rooms rocked my tilt-a-world head each time I staggered across the floor. No healthy-looking motherly glow for me; my *tout ensemble* consisted of a pickle-green face, reddened, road-map eyes, and over-stuffed ankles. Neither saltine crackers, prescription drugs, nor anything else alleviated the misery of my bub-bling caldron of soured stomach acid and my achy head.

After much pleading, my physician allowed me to take Dramamine for the nausea. Only then did I find any mea-sure of relief. I gave daily thanks at the altar of my simple desk job, hiding behind mounds of papers and books propped up in front of me. Not being able to keep my eye-lids open, I snoozed away oblivious to my surroundings.

Surely my supervisor observed my antics but found it easier to laugh and ignore me than fire me.

That entire winter I never donned normal-weight maternity clothes designed for colder weather. Oh, I wanted to wear them. In my sleepy repose, I dreamed about buying cute corduroy pleated tops with little bows and pretty ribbons, or wowing everyone in a sleek, demurely fitted pantsuit.

It didn't happen. I could not stand anything that added warmth to my body. From May through January, I dressed in light cotton, short-sleeved blouses, and thin skirts or slacks. Even then I suffered from normal room heat and my brewing, internal inferno. As the days and weeks progressed, I took on the appearance and ambling motion of a Sherman tank draped in damp attire that hung stoically from ample bulges.

I can laugh about it now, especially remembering my husband and our bedroom. I controlled the thermostat at night, and it never ever strayed above 60 degrees. He complained to anyone who would listen he might freeze to death before the baby arrived. I felt too bad to offer him sympathy.

Still, he found great sport in referring to me as "hot mama", but not because I acted particularly amorous in the bedroom. Baby-doll-style pajamas adorned my barrel belly. I could only sleep (if you can call my fitful, crazed-woman repose "sleeping") with a light sheet over my body. A fan continuously blew on my skin. Why? Because nothing helped the toughest pregnancy symptom of all—when I went to bed, rolls of sweat cascaded down my neck, torso, legs, and toenails, soaking my clothes and anything near me. Each morning I crawled out of bed in self-defense, leaving behind a three-foot-wide swath of sweat on the mattress. My body didn't return to normal temperature regulation for twelve months after giving birth.

Many years later in 1990, I developed a serious, physical illness that looked as if it might never go away. My body revisited my former sweating, uncomfortable, aggravated persona. As I moved from room to room, my body broke out in a sticky, stinky ambiance. If I took a shower, I perspired afterwards and needed another bath before putting on clean clothes. Tired. Sick. Grouchy and grumpy. And the same old, sweaty symptom.

In 1998, I turned fifty; I should have been in menopause. For a while that summer, I scurried from air-conditioned house to air-cooled car and back. Uninvited weeds grew to spectacular heights in my flower beds. Thankfully, I rediscovered the wisdom of purchasing a lightweight, basic wardrobe in different colors according to the season.

Each successive year has afforded me better health. In 2006, my long-term illness abated entirely. Now I perspire less, enjoy more energy, and take fewer medications. My memory and cognitive skills have returned to sharper levels than I enjoyed twenty years ago.

"Don't you suffer with any menopause-related symptoms?"

Not really. Sometimes I get warm, but I maintain a wardrobe that suits me: loose garments for everyday and layered items for dressy occasions. I wear flat shoes and less hosiery. My hair stays short and easy to fix. No more sitting under hair dryers or standing at the sink hot-rolling shoulder-length hair for me.

"Okay. One more question. Does it bother you to be labeled as menopausal?"

Oh, surely you jest! Fewer hormones mean I shave my legs less often. And since I am retired with no job requirements or responsibilities to my grown children, I have more time for me, my husband, and some fun hobbies. I do sport a spare tire that makes me look atypical of a "hot mama," but I've joined the gym, and I figure I'll have that conquered soon, too.

It's a new day. Me? Unhappy with menopause? Nah. I'm fine.

Cinda Crawford

Wine Cooler

My trip back home was long awaited,
I crossed off every day.
The bus ride there was a delight,
air-conditioned, movies, back I lay.

Now this is the good way to travel,
no driving to worry about.
It even has a "potty" in back,
in case I'm not in drought.

I looked outside at passing trees,
and thought about my bags.
Maybe I should have packed a coat
'cause all I brought were summer rags.

The bus did stop at our road's end,
I saw my cousins there.
We embraced and I exclaimed,
"It sure is hot and fair!"

We did things every day outside,
and I melted bit by bit.

My cousin said "She is tough . . .
. . . she'll get over it!"

Our final day there was a tour,
an age-old winery place.
It ended in the basement cooler,
even then I could feel my face!

I hid behind a strange, big guy,
for if my cousin saw me,
he would have made a spectacle
for all the world to see.

I could feel his eyes on me,
I saw the look of laughter.
Here it comes, get out quick!
Or I'll hear it ever after.

It's too late, I heard a voice!
It bellowed in the basement.
"Only you, my cousin girl
could hot flash in cool encasement!"

Every single person there
looked around to see
who it was with menopause . . .
And bright red face—that's me!

All I could do was smile back,
at all the wine tour eyes.
Silence filled the echo room,
I must say something wise.

But mental-pause tiptoed in,
I couldn't find a word.

Instead, my mouth betrayed me, and
my words were like lemon curd!

"It's my menopause you see,
The heat has done me in.
My cousin put me on the spot
And now I'll need some gin!"

Up the stairs I climbed as quick,
as my swollen legs could go,
and in the wake of my flying skirt,
they laughed a "HO HO HO!"

Glady Martin

Half a Mile from Hades

At a young age, I learned that menopause is like living a half mile from hell. Please let me explain.

Whoever chose the color black for funeral attire was obviously not from the South, nor was the misguided fool who deemed it necessary for a Southern gentleman *never* to remove his jacket at any social function. Unfortunately, a funeral *is* a social function; I think those with twisted senses of humor die on purpose in July and August.

That's how I felt from where I stood as a young lad of thirteen on that brutal August day at the "Rest of Your Life" cemetery in Inferno, Mississippi. Standing alongside the sweating throng about to enter ninety-three-year-old widow Mrs. Ellie May Dolittle's soul to everlasting peaceful sleep, there seemed to be nothing funny at all, except for the fact that she had been left a widow as a result of an unfortunate fishing accident involving a John Deere and Jack Daniels.

I wish that in her last will and testament Miss Ellie, as she was called, would have been kind enough to leave us either some shade or a breeze or both, but neither was in existence that day. Heat waves rose from her stately gray casket that was adorned with a lovely spray of magnolia, pinecones, and roses and the most unusual swag of the Confederate flag. But these finishing touches were barely visible to many of us due to the waterfall of perspiration pouring from heads and drenching our Sunday go-to-meetin' clothes. Old men wheezed and gasped for what I was sure would be their last breaths. *How convenient; all we'll need is the medical examiner's signature and a sharpened shovel to get the two-for-one special from the local funeral home,* I thought. Old ladies fanned themselves with anything within reach as their makeup fell, along with their bobby-pin curls. The preacher was on the brink of heat exhaustion, barely able to raise the Bible over his head.

White Igloo ice chests filled with Piggly Wiggly RCs and homemade sweet tea circled the tiny tent that provided the only shade in the cemetery. That shade, I assumed, was meant for Miss Ellie, who certainly didn't need it anymore, and for members of her family who sat almost comatose in creaking wooden folding chairs as the sun continued beating down us like Katrina would decades later beat the coast. And all this was *way before* Al Gore and global warming.

Fortunately, due to local gun laws or lack thereof, preachers didn't give long-winded sermons at funerals when the temperature was above 120 degrees, so my family soon headed back to our Chevrolet that had, like us, been soaking up solar rays for far too long. I heard screams and yells from other cars as unsuspecting mourners grabbed chrome door handles, only to find their flesh sizzling like fatback in a cast-iron skillet.

When we were at a safe distance from the tent, I ripped off my jacket like it was on fire—and it probably was—then reluctantly entered that four-door furnace made by General Motors. The back of my thighs landed on the molten plastic seat and rendered what I'm sure was going to be third-degree burns. My sister cried in agony as her elbow touched the red-hot chrome of the ashtray on the door. My father said one of the two cuss words I've ever heard him utter as his hands gripped the hard blue plastic steering wheel, which left him scampering for his sweat-soaked white handkerchief that he used much in the same way Louis Armstrong does in concert. All the while, my mother sat surprisingly still.

We left the cemetery with the windows rolled down and the old air conditioner blowing in its vain attempt to cool things down a bit. *What could be worse?* I thought. Everyone was miserable, scorched to the bone, flesh sloughing off like wax from a Christmas candle. Then I saw my father's eyes in the rearview mirror. He looked absolutely terrified, and he was hardly ever terrified about anything, being the only doctor in a small Southern town. I turned to my sister and mouthed the words "better buckle up."

About the time our seat belts clicked, I heard a moan that began deep in my mother's chest. I also heard her new black shoes, closed toe with sensible heels that were purchased for the funeral, hit the metal underpinnings of the dashboard. When the shoes came off we, like Pavlov's dogs, knew what was about to happen.

The gold bracelets on my mother's wrists started clanging and jangling as she pulled her hair high on the top of her head in a futile attempt to keep it from touching her hormone-reddened neck. From my vantage point in the backseat I could not see her face, but I knew it was as red as the tomatoes in my grandfather's garden. When her flashes began to come in waves, starting at her head and shooting through the floorboards of the Chevy, I knew no one was safe inside the vehicle.

You would have thought we were in a hellfire and brimstone backwoods church due to incessant use of the "Mary, Mother of God" and "Jesus, have mercy" that were flying around that sweltering Chevrolet like very unhappy hornets. My father frantically directed every air conditioner vent toward her, yelling to us kids to bow our heads and pray for relief.

Just about this time, gold buttons started flying from the front seat, as did the funeral high heels, lipstick, and makeup. Next came the stockings that were peeled from her like a surgeon removing rubber gloves, followed by the ever-present girdle. All the while moans escalated to screams, talking in tongues and seizures of some sort. She was coming out of those clothes, and she didn't care who saw her!

Hell was visiting upon my mother yet another menopausal hot flash. I felt so sorry for her; she was already soaking wet after Miss Ellie's blistering send-off, but now a second wave of a Niagara Falls was cascading from the top of her head. There really should be a law against this sort of thing. It's cruel and very unusual punishment for an otherwise cheerful and happy belle of the South, loving mother, and garden club member.

Menopause is scary, *even* from the backseat.

Tommy Polk

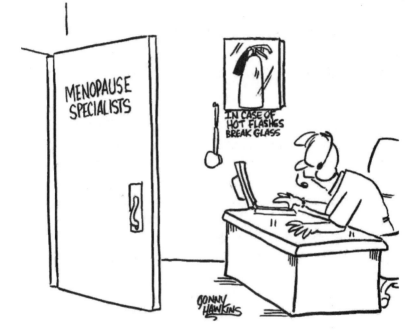

Highs and Lows

I was forty when I had a hysterectomy. My doctor told me that although my ovaries were intact, I might experience an early menopause and not to be concerned if I did. For the first six months or so, I was on full alert for any signs of "the change." When nothing happened, I forgot all about it.

It was not until my late forties when I found out what the word "hot flash" really meant. If you think you're having them, you're not. There's nothing flashy about them. In fact, they're closer to having someone stoke an internal Bessemer furnace. The heat begins with a warm glow in the solar plexus then builds in waves to scalding proportions and finally becomes nuclear at the hairline. Sweat drips, clothes darken, and if you're wearing more than one layer of clothes, you'll strip without shame—in the office, at church, wherever. That's what a hot flash is, and you'll know you are having them when you get to the point of giving them pet names. Mine were called "power surges."

Nights were worse than days. During the day, I was uncomfortable and sometimes embarrassed. At night, I would wake as the heat reached a crescendo, tossing off blankets no matter the temperature. The surges seemed to be on a schedule; I could count on waking at 2:00 AM and again at 6:30 AM. Who needs alarm clocks when you have your own personal fire-breathing dragon?

At a time when women complained that their husbands become distant and uninterested as they went through menopause, I had no such problem. During my hot flashes, my husband would look at me with sympathy. "Pretty bad, aren't they?" he would say as blush melted from my cheeks, and mascara ran down my face. "You're beautiful to me, and I love you." During my nighttime episodes, he would often rise and wet down a facecloth for me with cool water. He would replenish the water carafe next to my side of the bed every evening before we turned in for the night. And nearly every morning, my husband would cuddle close to me, and I would awake, my internal furnace on high, folded in his arms. It made me feel cherished, loved—and hot! I could never figure out how he stood it; it had to be like holding a jalapeño. But I would soon find out why.

We lived in Florida at the time, and the winter that year was unusually cold. We'd turned off the air conditioner in October and by late November, nighttime temperatures were plummeting into the forties and fifties. Not cold by the standards of most of the country, but South Florida winters are damp, not cold. The temperature changes come in the space of hours, not seasons.

I had gone for my annual checkup that January. My doctor had prescribed low-dose hormones to help me through my symptoms. My dragon was now only puffing smoke, and I was thrilled. I finally had control over my personal thermostat again! Well, most times anyway. It was often enough that I allowed color back into my wardrobe.

February was the coldest month, with daytime temperatures in the sixties and nights approaching the mid-thirties. Some mornings we had hoarfrost on the lawn. Early one morning I woke in my husband's arms and snuggled deeper, enjoying his warmth. I was glad that I didn't feel as though I was going to self-combust.

"Hon," my husband whispered in my ear, "do you think you could go off those pills for a while? Maybe just until spring?"

That was when I realized that the morning cuddle had less to do with sympathy than it did with my power surge. He had been warming himself at the furnace of my menopause before getting out of bed to start the day! I think it was the first pillow fight I had had since I was seven years old. There was no way I was letting the remark pass unnoticed. Besides, isn't menopause the advent of a second childhood anyway?

Kim A. Hoyo

Comforting Dreams

Dreams come true; without that possibility, nature would not incite us to have them.

John Updike

In 2003, my wife Scharre was diagnosed with breast cancer. After several consultations with her doctor and surgeon, she decided to have a double mastectomy even though the cancer was only detected in one breast. Scharre had the operation early in 2003 and spent the rest of that year undergoing chemotherapy.

When the chemotherapy was completed, Scharre was prescribed the drug Tamoxifen to be taken twice a day for five years. The oncologist explained that Tamoxifen reduced the amount of estrogen the body naturally produces; ten years earlier, in 1993, Scharre had had uterine cancer, resulting in a hysterectomy. She was also placed on hormone replacement therapy after her hysterectomy; the oncologist said that while the HRT she was taking did not cause her breast cancer, it appeared it may have accelerated the growth of these new cancer cells.

Since Scharre had been on HRT during her fifties, she

never experienced menopause. Now, at age sixty-some-thing, she learned that she would get to go through the "passage" after all, since the oncologist did not want to put her back on synthetic hormones. He warned Scharre that some of Tamoxifen's side effects included high-intensity hot flashes and night sweats.

After Scharre completely recovered from the effects of her chemotherapy treatments and was feeling back to normal, I asked her what she wanted to do to celebrate her survival from her second bout with cancer. Scharre replied that she would like to take another trip to Alaska with our truck and trailer, similar to the trip we had taken four years earlier. With that said, we made our plans and soon departed from our hometown of Crescent City, California, heading north to Alaska.

Both retired, Scharre and I love to camp comfortably, and do so in our twenty-six foot trailer, which has all the ameni-ties you could wish for. Excited about our trip, Scharre stocked up the trailer, anticipating our latest adventure. Every day brought a new twist in the road, but we were enjoying ourselves immensely, with the exception of Scharre's menopausal flare-ups. I felt sorry for her when this happened and as any good husband would do, I made sure she was comfortable, then I stayed out of her way.

The night sweats were the worst part of her symptoms. Several times a night I would wake up to find Scharre on top of the covers naked, covered in sweat, and miserable. The amazing part of this was that it would be in the low thirties, but she was on fire. She would eventually recover from these hot flashes—as she cooled down, the sweat on her body would begin to dry, and she would get cold. Scharre would then pull all the covers off of me trying to get warm!

While we were camping at Denali National Park in Alaska, we attended several fireside talks where the rangers gave detailed instructions on what to do if a bear attacked. After one particularly rattling bear-related fireside talk, we cautiously walked back in the dark to our campsite and went to bed. Snoozing away nice and warm in our bed, I had a crazy dream; I was at a tourist attraction, and they had hired teenagers to identify fresh bear scat on the property so they knew where to take tourists to see the bears. I ended up alone in a cart being pulled by a small garden tractor, and legendary entertainer Johnny Carson was the driver.

Johnny drove the tractor down this dirt road, which had brush on both sides. After going a short distance, both of us could see dirt being thrown up over the top of the brush beside the road. Johnny pulled up next to the area and it became evident to both of us that a bear was behind the brush, and it was a big bear. It then became immediately apparent to me that I was in a vulnerable position if the bear came at us; I was debating whether to stand my ground, go into a fetal position, or try to outrun both Johnny and the bear.

In the real world outside my crazy dream, Scharre was recovering from one of her hot flashes. Becoming quite chilled, she quietly crawled out of bed and picked up the big feather tick comforter from the couch. At the exact instance I was anticipating the bear's charge at Johnny and me, Scharre threw the heavy comforter onto the bed and on top of me.

Luckily we were in an RV park—we had to visit the Laundromat the next day to wash our sheets. I've had my own night sweats ever since.

Cliff Johnson

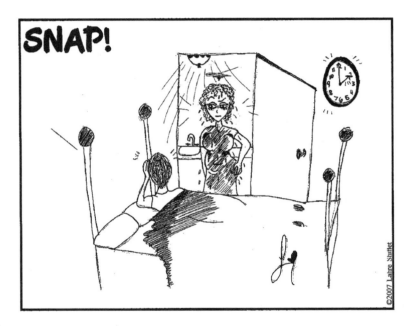

"Why in the world would you take a shower at two AM?"

Flashes of Hope

One leg escapes, coolness sought,
Wide awake with no clear thought.
One AM, now two, then four,
"Oh Lord," I pray, sliding to the floor.

The window's cracked and so am I
Such internal heat, it makes me cry.
Endless days and sleepless nights,
Cranky kids and spousal fights.

Gazing at me with puzzled looks,
This woman who no longer cooks.
The boiling pot is now inside,
The outer me feels ten feet wide.

My girlish form on a slippery slope
One more loss as I try to cope.
Mountaintop joys and valley lows,
Minute to minute one never knows.

Tiptoeing around, my family tries
To feed me with unending lies;

"It's okay, honey," or "You look great."
"I love you, Mom," but it's too late.

They try to help as I moan and groan
"Why can't they just leave me alone?"
My heart skips a beat as away I run,
I believe a heart attack has begun.

Another trip to my doctor's side
With a smile she tries so hard to hide.
Another daft patient with phantom fear,
The haggard old lady I see in the mirror.

How about a diet or a hormone cream?
I'll try them all as I continue to dream
Of the second half of this crazy life,
The changeover along with the strife.

A more confident me, with mood swings calm,
Walking on a beach, sitting under a palm.
Yes it will happen, I am woman, I am strong,
Believe it with me as we journey along.

Menopausal women together we'll survive
Sharing our options, adrift, but alive,
For now I am tired, no time to recap,
We'll talk later, I need a nap!

Judy Quick Anderson

8

THE NEW ME

One thousand days to learn; ten thousand days to refine.

Japanese Proverb

A Half Century Yet to Go

*Age is a question of mind over matter. If you
don't mind, it doesn't matter.*

Satchel Paige

The gifts were strewn as if at a child's party. But I was
no child. I had turned fifty years old and was feeling worse
than old. I felt ancient. The cake was covered with so
many candles its bright heat almost burned me. As I
strained to blow them out in one breath to show I was still
full of life, the guests cheered for me as if I had won my
way into some kind of secret order. If I had, I didn't want
to be a member. An over-the-hill club was definitely not
my idea of special.

Why was this so hard for me? Why did I feel a sense of
grief, a longing for that good, young age of forty or, better
yet, thirty? I balked at those birthdays, too, as each made
me feel I was losing my youth and had nothing to show
for it. But none had made me so sad and weary as this one.

Making my way around the room, I watched my friends
laughing and chatting with each other. Most of them were
in their fifties. A few had yet to reach this milestone, but

several others were in their "golden years." They seemed to have survived this rite of passage with grace and even a bit of humor.

Don't they realize their lives are more than half over? Don't they know that career dreams, if not already realized, are most likely unattainable? Couldn't they see themselves—necks wobbling like turkeys, hands spotted and knobby, breasts sagging, tummies bulging, hair bright with bottle-color, eyes needing glasses?

And here I now stand, one of them.

"Bodies are boring," my mother once told me. "They always need something." I'm beginning to understand her statement.

Snippets of conversation reach me.

"I'm working on a book."

"I'm walking two miles every morning."

"I've gone back to college."

Curiously, these women don't feel their lives are almost over but, rather, just beginning—again.

Even though most look middle-aged, incredibly, they seem to love it. They look like women—not girls, of course, but vital, interesting, and interested women—full of life and sparkling with the enjoyment of who they are and what their lives bring them.

Some are still quite beautiful. Many have suffered devastating losses—husbands, siblings, and, worst of all, children. Others fight enormous health battles. They put on their wigs, cover their bandages, then head out to party, to laugh and seek joy in life.

Suddenly, I envisioned an entire new chapter of freedom in my life, with time to discover new interests and pursue them. I had a delicious feeling of stepping to the top of the hill and surveying all that lies beyond, just waiting for me to explore as lightly or as deeply as I desire. And there would be no more responsibilities, except those I willingly took on, such as spending quality time with my husband, children, grandchildren, and mother.

With health on my side, I can climb mountains, walk in the surf, or play tennis, or golf, dominoes, or bridge. I can volunteer at church, hospitals, or homeless shelters, take classes at the local community college, write a book, sing in the choir, learn country line dancing, prepare gourmet meals, travel to foreign lands. The possibilities are endless. Life begins at fifty? No. It just gets better, richer, more precious, exciting.

Depressed? Not anymore. I joined in the laughter and fun and enjoyed the celebration of the anniversary of my birth.

I have lived half a century. Amazing.

Jean Stewart

Fifty Already?

Of my two score years and ten
fifty feels a lot like plenty.
Aching back and knees that creak,
appetite's hearty, memory's weak.

The law I've always held so dear
is strongly pulling at my rear.
How can a citizen like me
defy the law of gravity?

Each day I face the mirror, undaunted,
to count more chins than I ever wanted.
My hair's a youthful brown, it's true.
Does she or doesn't she? You bet I do!

Different glasses, near and far,
help me read or drive a car.
And so I don't succumb to ills
I start each morning downing pills.

But life's not over, not by half.
I handle changes with a laugh.
I'm still myself, and I'd feel nifty
if I could get over turning fifty.

June Williams

Granny Pants

If you obey all the rules, you miss all the fun.

Katharine Hepburn

I swore that it would never happen to me, but it has. I have become the nightmare of my teenage years. I have grayed, and bits of me that were once taut are now wiggly and jiggly, and bits of me that used to be loose have frozen up. This I have borne with relative good grace. But today I became my own *bête noire*.

I have worn all kinds of jeans in my life. In the seventh grade I had elephant bell hip-huggers that were more patch than pant and were they ever cool! I cut the seams out of the jeans and put in a big triangle of brightly colored material. I wanted to do this myself and wear them to the Sadie Hawkins dance. I couldn't sew, and my mom wasn't going to be home in time, so I tried some good old Elmer's glue. That didn't work so well, so I stapled them and called it good. I went over to my friend's house. "Wow, Liz! Look at your jeans!" What I heard was, "Your jeans are so cool."

"Mom," my friend said, "look at Liz's jeans."

"I bet you did those all by yourself, didn't you?" her mom asked me.

"Yes ma'am, I did," I said not too modestly.

"Would you like me to just give them a quick going-over so your staples don't show so much?" Since one of the staples was, at that very moment, jabbing itself painfully into my calf, I agreed. Her mother fixed my pants with a needle and thread.

In high school I wore my jeans way, way, way too long so that the cuff would get appropriately frayed and dirty. In the '80s I wore super-tight jeans in every color of the rainbow—the tighter and brighter the better, to go with my enormous shoulder pads and gigantic hair.

Then I had a decade or so when I just could not find any jeans that both fit and looked right. Until yesterday. I tried on a pair of jeans and asked my daughter if she thought they were too short. "Don't worry, Mom. Nobody will notice," she replied. Uh-oh. I started to fret and tried to see my reflection in a glass door. And then her words, "Nobody will notice," sank in, and I had an epiphany: *Nobody will notice me!*

I was determined to find a pair of jeans that *someone* would notice. But after a long day of trying on pair after pair of jeans at store after store, I was ready to give up. I had tried on jeans that snapped just below where my bosom currently resides. I tried on jeans that snapped way, way, way lower than that. I tried on jeans that were belled and boot cut, and tapered. I tried on jeans that were "relaxed" and jeans I suspected of being on the verge of a breakdown. I tried on jeans that were the deep, new indigo and rejected them as dorky, and I tried on jeans that looked like they had been worn by an auto mechanic for a few weeks. I think I tried on every pair of jeans in the greater metropolitan area.

And then I found them—the perfect pair. I might have

bought myself one of those "Queen of Denial" T-shirts too, because I was definitely doing some fast self-talk. The only reason I even tried them on was because they were on sale. I'm a sucker for something on sale. But I loved them! They were almost as comfortable as scrub pants. I preened in front of the mirror. *These look like something Katharine Hepburn would wear, I thought. So neat looking, so flattering, and so comfortable. Are they a little short though? Nah! I see people wearing their britches all different lengths. They're fine. And sooooo comfortable!*

Why were they so comfortable? I am going to tell you something now that I never, ever thought I would say in a million, billion years. They had a half-elastic waist. And long, loose legs. And square, sailor-style pockets. And I loved them. And they were not Katharine Hepburn pants. They were not sailor pants. They were Granny Pants, pure and simple.

Today, I am free! Liberated! Released through the sheer perseverance in surviving this long from the dictates of fashion! I can wear any darned thing I want to wear and nobody notices! Goodbye, panty hose; hello, knee socks! Fair-thee-well, heels, and howdy-doo, driving moccasins! Hasta la vista, cuffs and collars and waistbands, and hello to the wonderful world of jersey knits! Katharine Hepburn, my hind leg! Hello, Granny Pants!

Elizabeth Sowdal

Momentarily Mature

Cherish all your happy moments; they make a
fine pin cushion for old age.

Booth Tarkington

My skin and various other body parts tell a different story, but at heart, I never aged beyond eighteen years old. In my fifties, I still liked to be silly, wonder, change my image daily, cop an attitude, laugh out loud, make faces, make fun, and drive fast.

Then menopause crept up on me like a big shadowy cat, toying with me, and swiping at me with hot flashes and mood swings without ever showing itself. The shadow-cat curled around me, creating a fog of sadness. At first, I attributed my sadness to the fact that my late-in-life child had found his independence in a driver's license and car of his own. But then things got worse.

Somewhere along my way, I had lost my sense of humor. Getting the wrong angle with my home barista machine and spraying steamed milk all over the ceiling and cabinets made me think of how hard it was going to be to clean it up, not of how funny it would be to see if I could do it again. My Labrador's romp through the mud puddles and spray caused by a broken soak hose caused concern about his dirty paw prints, instead of making me want to join him or even just laugh at him.

For once, I didn't try to excuse joint pain as a result of wrestling with the dog or assume it was that old skiing injury. The bad photos of me were no longer just a glitch in the digital formatting of the camera or that dratted wide-angle lens. Only barely making out the headlines in the newspaper wasn't because of the ink blurring in the printing process, a mystically common occurrence it had seemed.

I should have known something long term and serious was happening when Halloween, my favorite holiday, came to our house with no candles in pottery pumpkins and no fake spider webs appearing on the front porch. Normally reveling in the excuse for many forms of chocolate on hand, the cooler weather, the fun of costumes and pretend personas without the burden of expected gifts, I almost forgot it was October 31. The woman who had scared, or at least impressed, trick-or-treaters with a witch hat and a green Avon-Cucumber-Facial complexion, was watching television with the porch light out.

The worst thing was that I didn't even realize what was happening. We all have down times, so I just bumbled through day after day not realizing that I was chemically saddened by my own traitor hormones. Estrogen had turned to terrorism and didn't send a videotape claiming responsibility.

Because I complained of constant headaches, my friend took me to my doctor. My doctor never said the word "menopause," probably thinking I'd have to be a real simpleton not to know what all these symptoms were about. He did, however, say the word "depression" and gave me a temporary low dose of antidepressants.

It didn't take long. December brought a magical snow-storm to our hillside home. My high-school-senior son noticed it starting about 10:00 PM with intricate, feathery flakes and suggested we take our four-wheel drive to the top of the hill to check it out up there. The first symptom that I was becoming myself again was my running out the door without a coat, right behind him, slipping and gig-gling and not even thinking about how really stupid it was to embark on such a trip.

It was magical. Snowflake fog surrounded us as he slowly drove the winding climb. Trees were shadowy skeletons floating in smoky white flakes, the road almost covered and completely trackless. The snow was sticking! Oh, joy! The car even slid a little at the steeper curves. We stopped at the top where the forest service had gated off the rest of the road as it turned to gravel. There the forest was white, silent, and dizzying as we looked straight up through the open sunroof.

I felt eighteen again (and my son really was eighteen) so there was no grown-up around to remind us that we needed to head back down the hill before conditions became more dire. Steep downhill grades, slick curvy roads, and gravity can challenge even a four-wheel drive with studded snow tires.

We turned at the forest service gate and started back home, still happily oblivious to the potential peril. The road was less steep at the top so the realization that the snow had accumulated significantly only made the adventure better. We could barely see the tracks we'd made coming up. The tires on the snow made that crunchy squeak, not even touching roadbed.

My "way cool" was followed by an "uh-oh" as my son lightly braked at the first real hill, only to realize it wouldn't do much good. Deftly, he slipped the car, already in four-wheel drive, into the lowest gear. Creeping around the curves, he gently countered little skids, hands firm on the top of the steering wheel, eyes squinting close to the windshield. We could see little except snow in the air and snow packed on the road, but knew the barely visible trees marked the edge of a couple of pretty steep banks.

"Uh-oh," I repeated, but he was still smiling, calm and confident, so I slowly let out the breath I'd been holding.

Not only did we survive our foolishness without having to call a tow truck, but I learned I could feel joy again. And at the same time, my youngest made it clear he had become a competent, if not particularly cautious, almost-adult.

I survived "the change." We survived the adventure. Life is good again. Maybe better.

Sallie Brown

Red-Hot Mama

If you have a lemon, make lemonade.

Howard Gossage

Twenty years ago, my idea of being a "red-hot mama" would probably have included stiletto heels, a black lace bustier, and a twenty-foot boa—the kind with feathers, not a forked tongue. I picture myself strutting around a stage, doing a bit of a bump and grind, while giving the men my come-hither look.

In real life, I would never have cavorted around like an exotic dancer, even in the privacy of my own bedroom, let alone on a stage. I'm a lot more comfortable in flats than heels, my industrial-strength bras don't have a lace ruffle in sight, and the only feathers I'm use to swinging are at the end of a duster. Still, it's nice to have that sexy image of myself tucked away in a deep, dark corner of my mind.

Now that I'm having an intimate relationship with menopause, the words "red-hot mama" have an entirely different connotation. Forget the stilettos, bustier, and boa. Substitute memory loss, sweat, and support hose, and you'll have a better idea of my real life. I'd like to say

I'm not complaining, but I am. *Loudly.* And repeatedly. I may be entering menopause and the last large chunk of my life before I'm hauled off to do the bump and grind in the Great Hereafter, but I am not going quietly.

I don't mind getting older and wiser on the journey of life, particularly the wiser part. I just don't like the current stretch of road I'm on at the moment. But having chosen not to take the hormone detour, I've decided to tough it out along the scenic route. But I do have a few tricks up my sleeve to make the journey a little smoother. Make that a short sleeve. Better yet, sleeveless.

I've started using soy milk in my morning oatmeal, hoping my body has read the same articles that I have about Japanese women having an easier menopause, partly due to their higher consumption of soy products. Or was that sushi? Teriyaki? Wasabi? No, I'm pretty sure it was soy. Besides, putting hot, green paste-like wasabi on oatmeal would be more likely to start a fire than to put one out.

I joined a gym, hired a personal trainer, and work out three times, okay, twice a week because exercise is supposed to help with hot flashes. However, catching sight of myself in the mirror with a fire engine–red complexion and sweat pouring down my face is less than encouraging. I've had to reassure a number of people at my gym that I'm not having a heart attack. The staff keeps a close eye on me, and everyone at the front desk knows my name.

And I chug water by the bottle, hoping to drown those pesky free radicals that cause aging, while flushing the toxins out of my body. Darn. Why did I have to go and say the flush word? Just a minute while I answer nature's call. The old bladder isn't what it used to be either.

I'm back.

Where was I in my long list of complaints? There's something else I wanted to say. Something about . . . got it. My memory. My once reliable memory has transformed from a steel trap to Swiss cheese. Not only does new information no longer enter my brain for more than ten seconds, but the old stuff is leaving—possibly looking for a cooler climate. Why I can no longer remember my phone number, but can still recite the formula for determining the circumference of a circle, I'll never understand.

On the bright side, partial memory loss isn't all bad. It's nice to meet new people again—for the fourth or fifth time. And if you're talking to me, you don't have to worry if you've told me that story before. I'm not going to remember. Unfortunately, this is a two-way street, and I've been known to repeat the same story. Repeat the same story.

While I'm sitting in front of the fan with a cold compress on my chest and a chocolate brownie in my hand, I console myself with the thought that menopause is shorter than puberty. If I made it through the first, I can certainly make it through the second.

When I do hit the other side of menopause, watch out, world. I might go out and buy myself some stilettos. I just hope I can fit my orthopedic insoles in them.

Harriet Cooper

Old Is New Again

*Years may wrinkle the skin, but to give up inter-
est wrinkles the soul.*

General Douglas MacArthur

Sure, I already had a degree in finance; it was for security reasons that I studied the field in the first place. You
know, that job-stability thing. Yet, it was the end of the
last decade of the twentieth century, and I felt it was time
for a change.

I was about to turn fifty and suddenly wanted an
adjustment, a change in the direction of the wind and the
aromas that filtered through my nose. So what if I had job
seniority and worked independently. Office pungency
had become offensive. I needed to smell the roses—roses
with my name on them. So I quit my job.

No, I did not just up and quit. I planned it. In the early
nineties, I had gone back to school and studied communi-
cation, English, and art history. I started collecting writing
samples early, saved some money, and set up a timetable,
all for a metamorphosis from old to new. My friends
thought I was crazy. Quit a good job? Why not? Everything

I ever wanted was screaming at me to go for it.

To prove I was not playing around, I threw a success party the summer before I quit. I invited everyone I knew—friends and enemies—to come celebrate my stepping out. As in a debutante ball, I introduced myself to the world as an up-and-coming journalist. No longer would I have to keep up with accounting stats or economic trends.

Only there was a catch. I was not only coming of age as a journalist, I was also maturing. Maturing in the way most women do not think about until it slaps us in our faces and the rest of our bodies for that matter: hair loss, sagging skin, bifocal glasses, mood swings, forgetfulness, night sweats, fake signs of heart attacks—you name it, I experienced it. Menopause. All the planning in the world did not prepare me for this passage. Besides, it didn't fit with being a creative writer.

Realizing that menopause was amending my plan, I made adjustments. Instead of becoming down in the mouth, I set out to make "the change" work for me. I blamed all my errors on it. When I forgot to keep an appointment with friends I simply said, "I'm going through menopause. You know, I have a hard time remembering anything." If I became curt with anyone, I blamed it on being menopausal. When the mood pendulum was swinging from east to west, from my mouth would come, "You know how it is when you're going through the change." Yes, it worked, and it continues to do so. Everybody understands, and nobody complains; they sympathize. In turn, I get to set any schedule I want, change my mind when I choose, even cry for no reason because everyone accepts me. Mother Nature is to blame for my idiosyncrasies, not me.

This current life of mine is rewarding, but fluctuations play their part. Yet, in hindsight, if I had it to do all over, I would still proceed to design the "new" me. It is not about becoming rich and famous. It is about enjoying life like you never have before, in doing what you have always dreamed of doing and loving it—with all its consequences.

I now write as a career choice, carry an AARP card in my wallet, and never felt better than I do now. Just think, if I had kept my secure career job, I would still have nine years to work before I could do what I do now. A transformation and "the change" never felt so good.

Sylvia McClain

Keep Your Chin Up!

*I believe that sometimes you have to look reality
in the eye and deny it.*

Garrison Keillor

Turning fifty was bad enough, but one day over brunch,
my friend said, "Honey, have you ever considered a face-
lift?" I knew I couldn't ignore this aging thing any longer.

So I trotted to my therapist to sort out the newest chapter in my life—to talk about the skin slipping off my lower
face like Jell-O sliding off a plate. Walking into her office, I
noticed puffiness, redness, and bruises on her face.

"Have you been in an accident?" I asked, worried.

"Oh no!" she said. "I had a face-lift."

Great, I thought. *Here's my role model for aging, and even she
gets a face-lift.* I felt betrayed.

The obsession with the sagging lower jowl ballooned.
Some women obsess over thighs, hips, and behinds, but
not me. It was the face, and not just the face. It was the
skin around and south of my mouth. *Did it sag when someone looked down? How much? Did they have those little pleats in
their skin like I did?*

I'd stand in front of the mirror, pull the skin taut behind my ears, and look twenty years younger. *Maybe I could tape it?* Then I'd rub on expensive moisturizing creams with promises of tighter, more youthful skin, but the pleats still greeted me each morning.

"Don't worry, Mom," my daughter said. "It's the genes. But I'm sure glad I take after Dad's family."

Tuesdays became a challenge. A small local produce store advertised: *Every Tuesday, all seniors fifty-five and older get a 10-percent discount.* I hadn't noticed the huge white banner with gigantic red letters until the day the cashier gave me a 10-percent discount—without asking.

How dare they! I called my eighty-two-year-old aunt in Indiana and lamented, "The cashier at the store just gave me a senior discount, and I'm not even fifty-five!"

I was fifty-four, and no one was giving me a senior discount one year early. I just knew it was my sagging face.

For a few weeks, I avoided shopping at that store on Tuesdays. Then I contrived a plan: Each week, I'd secretly select the checkout cashier. *Was the cashier male or female? Young or old? Would that person think I was fifty-five?*

I made sure my makeup and hair looked good. I avoided turtlenecks because they emphasized the sag. I'd approach the cashier, hold my head as high as possible to keep the skin from sagging, smile, and mentally dare them to give me that dreaded discount.

For a few weeks this worked, and I'd march out of the store feeling victorious and young. No 10-percent discount on my receipt!

One Tuesday, I picked a tall, lanky kid who looked young enough to be my son. *Shouldn't be a problem,* I thought. As he scanned the fresh produce, I noticed his eyes scanning my face. *This is the real test.* I held my head higher. Without a word, he punched that dreaded code: 10-percent discount!

"Dangity, dang, dang," I muttered as I studied my receipt. *What went wrong?*

This time I didn't race in the house, call my aunt, fall on my bed in tears, or smash my mirror. Putting my groceries away, part of a familiar Bible verse came to mind: "Though outwardly we are wasting away...."

Great, I thought, *it's obvious to everyone that I'm wasting away.*

"Help me, God," I sighed, "to age graciously, even in Southern California where everyone seems to have face-lifts."

Don't believe for a moment that I'm not tempted to get a face-lift, and maybe I will. Until then, I practice what my mother taught me: Hold your head up high and keep your chin up.

Jeanne Pallos

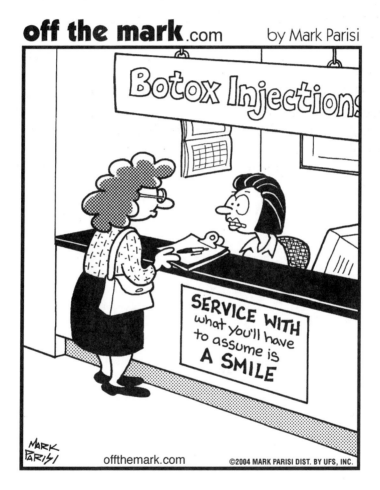

Reprinted by permission of Off the Mark and Mark Parisi. ©2004 Mark Parisi.

Midlife Lift!

Flabby thighs?
Exercise.

Belly bulge?
Don't indulge.

Hairy lip?
Wax and rip.

Wrinkled skin?
Collagen.

Tummy flap?
Herbal wrap.

Mouth obscure?
Botox cure.

Bosom slant?
Breast implant.

Tush amuck?
Liposuck.

Best repair?
Grin and bear!

Beverly Spooner

Middle-Aged Blues

*You can dance anywhere if you can dance in
your mind, in your heart.*

Jacques D'Amboise

I first noticed that Father Time and Mother Nature were
creeping up behind me when I was about thirty-five years
old. I began to see more highlights in my hair, compli-
ments of Father Time rather than my hairdresser. I also
began to see a change in my face. Gone was the glow of
youth, and a sallow skin tone replaced my once peachy-
pink complexion. I began to fight these frightening recog-
nitions with more frequent trips to the hairdresser to
camouflage my natural highlights and to the department
store to buy jars of goo that would help diminish my
washed-out skin tone.

Unfortunately, as Father Time and Mother Nature
marched on, so did my problems. Slowly, things began to
change. Things that made me realize I was getting old.
Getting out of the shower one day and preparing to go to
work resulted in an astonishing revelation; my once-
perky breasts had now become an awning for my feet.

And speaking of feet, where did they go? I only see them now when I'm lying down. And talking about lying down, guess where one's sloping chest lands when you lie on your back? My underarms now have their own pillows! Trips to the department store to expand my wardrobe revealed a clothing conspiracy against ample-size, forty-plus women. During one recent trip, I received a warm greeting from the salesclerk; she looked all of twelve years old and weighed all of six pounds. She asked if she could help me with my clothing selection.

"Who keeps putting size-fourteen tags on size-eight clothes?" was my first question. Miss Six Pounds responded that perhaps the clothes did not fit because of the cut or style. *Who cut them? Barbie?* I thought. *Barbie and a number-two pencil are the only two things I know of that have a waist that small.*

Miss Six Pounds graciously escorted me to the plus-size department and selected outfits that were big enough to cover a car. "Thank you, no!" I said. "I'm not a size eight, but I'm also not an Oldsmobile."

Reminders of my middle-aged blues journey also surface when I make my yearly jaunt to see my gynecologist. A recent trip made me feel really ancient as I was greeted by another twelve-year-old who updated my file. Miss Twelve-Year-Old then escorted me to the examination room. I donned my paper gown and waited for my doctor to arrive.

"How are you, Karen? Having any problems?" he asked.

"Well, my monthly cycle is now semi-monthly. My PMS is worse, and my body temperature always seems to be at least 101 degrees."

My doctor replied with a *"Hmmmnnnnn"* and looked at my records. "Karen, I see you are forty-eight years old now; you do realize that you have reached a time in your life where your body will be going through changes."

"When will these changes stop?" I asked.

"Never," the doctor responded, "you will just have to get used to them."

"Isn't there a pill, or vitamin, or herb or something I can take to feel better?"

"No, not really," the doctor replied. "Vitamins and herbs won't hurt you, but we really haven't come up with a good solution for helping women at this particular crossroads in their lives."

Dressed-up words that translated to: *You're old, sweetheart, deal with it!* Why, did I suddenly feel like Helen Hayes? *Crossroads? What crossroads?* As the doctor exited, and I trashed their designer paper gown, smiling Miss Twelve-Year-Old reappeared with a prescription and free samples of Geritol and Metamucil.

"Here you are, ma'am, maybe these will make you feel better. Would you like me to stick these samples in your bag?"

Resisting the urge to tell her where to stick them, I bit my tongue, flashed my show-biz smile and responded with the affirmative.

Leaving the doctor's office, I stopped at the cafe in his building to ponder my fate. I purchased a Diet Pepsi and discarded the Geritol and Metamucil. As I made my way to a table, I quickly glanced at the other customers in the cafe. No twelve-year-olds! No Barbies! Just regular folks sitting down eating and drinking. What fun!

These other customers provided me with a reprieve from feeling like a worn-out piece of elastic. I started to think about the good, the bad, and the ugly times of my life. *Do I really want to be twelve years old again?* I don't think so! *Do I really want to look like a number-two pencil?* No, that might make it hard to figure out which way to put on my clothes. I realized that age really was irrelevant. It's attitude that's important.

Father Time and Mother Nature are going to keep marching regardless of how much I whine. I realized it was time to go find an eighteen-hour Playtex something-or-another to hoist up whatever is sloping toward my feet, put it on, and march along with Father Time and Mother Nature—enjoying the moments as they are given to me.

Karen Gaebelein

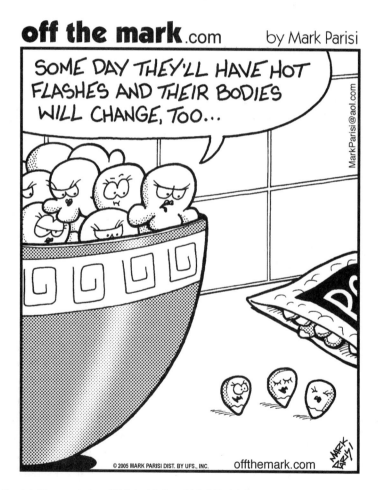

Reprinted by permission of Off the Mark and Mark Parisi. ©2005 Mark Parisi.

Indian Summer

In the spring of my young life, I wouldn't have dreamed of having to worry about something called a monthly curse or recurring tummy aches that could send me straight to bed. I wouldn't have dreamed of having to worry if I wore white pants, except that I might get grass stains on my knees. I wouldn't ever have turned down a chance to go swimming, and I wouldn't have carried a bunch of "supplies" in my purse, just in case. It was good to be a child free of such worries.

I remember as an adolescent thinking the classroom I was sitting in had turned into a glowing furnace. I could feel my face turning red, from the heat in my body rather than from the shyness that had previously brightened my cheeks. After class, I recall standing in front of the mirror in the girls' restroom, raising my arms to adjust my ponytail. I felt embarrassed and confused by unfamiliar wet stains under both arms of my lavender cotton blouse.

Thirty-eight years later, knocking on the door marked "menopause," I wondered why that same furnace, the one that had etched itself on my memory in adolescence, had fired up again. Instead of the underarms of my lavender blouse being soaked, my whole body was drenched. They say guys sweat and girls glow. My glow was a power surge. I learned to compensate for these frequent surges by wearing lighter blouses, by never wearing sweaters, by kicking the covers off at night, and by pretending I was vacationing in a lovely, but humid, tropical paradise. My husband compensated by scooting away when the tropical paradise created by my body heat threatened his good night's sleep.

When my mother went through menopause, there was a stereotype of midlife. Older women were painted as unattractive and asexual. We boomers grew up in a time of plenty, a time of bigger, better, and more, and we universally adopted a belief that we could have it all. We think it's our right to stay young forever, while at the same time saying we accept ourselves as we are. These notions are fed by today's television shows, movies, and magazines, which depict the menopausal woman as youthful, sexy, vibrant, and active.

We've dyed, tucked, stretched, and firmed our way into hanging onto our youth. We wonder in amazement how our children got to be as old as we are. A baby-boomer friend recently pondered, "If my son is thirty-five, how old am I? I don't think of myself as being a day over thirty!"

I attend a water aerobics class filled with nearly forty women ranging in age from fifty to eighty-something. Many have traveled the world, studied, and earned degrees that they didn't have time for when they were raising children. Most have added plump curves to their bodies since adolescence, cozy nests that little grandchildren and great-grandchildren love to snuggle into on a regular basis. These girls accept their mature curves, but stretch and tone to keep their joints mobile, their hearts and lungs healthy, and their bones strong. They have a zest for life. In that swimming pool, I hear more talk about sex or good-looking lifeguards than I do about menopause and more talk about trips, classes, and projects than about aches and pains. Some show up steadied by canes or supported by walkers, but when they get into the water, their spirits aren't a day over sixteen.

One thing has changed since adolescence. As a teenager, I knew everything, *absolutely everything*. Menopause has left me smarter than I felt just a few years ago. Fluctuating hormones used to wreak havoc not only with my moods, but also with my ability to think clearly. The fog has lifted. I feel pretty smart again, but still not as smart as I felt as a teenager, when I knew more than *anyone* over thirty.

Another thing has changed. When I was an adolescent, the boys I noticed in my class were what we now call "stud-muffins." Today, a lot of those same *boys* with their potbellies and balding heads resemble muffins that have expanded over the tops of their baking tins. Those very characteristics now make them cute grandpas, laughing boyishly and enjoying life with their friends, adult children, and grandkids.

As a baby boomer, I was blessed with hormone-replacement therapy, just what I believed I deserved to stay young and protected from aging. Then someone pulled the rug out from under me and took away my estrogen, leaving me wondering how I could stay young while dealing with a drop in hormone production. But, like puberty, menopause is a natural process, and I found ways to get through it.

As summer becomes fall, I pause to bask in the warm colors of the Indian summer of my life. I enjoy who I am today, and I look forward to knowing the person I will become in my winter days. Today, I play with my grandkids while the crunchy leaves drop from our big oak tree and I get grass stains on the knees of my white jeans.

Pat Nelson

Blessed Indeed

When you make the finding yourself—even if you're the last person on earth to see the light— you'll never forget it.

Carl Sagan

"Get out of the way! I'm having a flash!" Mom hollered as she yanked the freezer door open and fanned herself with a package of pork chops.

Of course, like any other kid, I giggled at this spectacle until my sides ached.

"Just wait, little Miss Smarty Pants," she snapped. "Someday you'll realize that hot flashes aren't very darned funny!"

Crow's feet, white hair, and thickening eyeglasses were outward signs that Mom was getting older. But the "Big M" (as Dad and I jokingly called menopause) caught everyone off guard. Overnight, my mild-mannered mother turned into an achy, cranky bundle of nerves. Her futile attempts to cool off during frequent meltdowns transformed our cozy home into an igloo.

Usually sharp as a tack, Mom became absentminded

after the Big M moved in. She forgot names, dates, and phone numbers, and continually misplaced her car keys only to find them in crazy places like her underwear drawer. She'd wake up with a jolt at 3:30 AM remembering she'd left laundry hanging on the clothesline, or she'd realize, as Dad and I were spitting peas into our napkins, that she seasoned them with sugar instead of salt.

No doubt about it, the Big M was scary business.

Like most teenage girls, I didn't spend a lot of time worrying about the pitfalls of becoming elderly. I lived in the moment, certain that youth, beauty, and a fresh, uncluttered mind would last forever. And for a number of years I was blissfully unbothered by the fact that my biological clock was ticking away. Then, without warning, the young woman in the mirror was kidnapped by a thief in the night who replaced the smooth-skinned, unlined image in the glass with a face that would never again be mistaken for twenty-one.

It was all downhill from there.

The outward signs of advancing age began hitting me so fast that it was difficult to keep up with them all. One day my eye doctor informed me that I needed bifocals just hours after I discovered a large colony of white hairs that had suddenly invaded my scalp like one of the seven plagues of Egypt.

And a few weeks later on the morning of my fortieth birthday, I ordered a cup of coffee at McDonald's and the little whippersnapper behind the counter charged me the senior citizen price. I was stunned for a moment, not sure if I should get upset or pretend it never happened.

It wasn't long before Mother Nature delivered her next punch. I woke up from a sound sleep, threw back the covers, and stood gasping in front of a fan as sweat drizzled down my chest and back. Even in my groggy state of mind, I knew I wasn't simply overheated. The Big M had arrived. And with every hot flash, I lost a little piece of my mind. Just like Mom, I forgot people's names that I'd known for years, blanked when reciting phone numbers, and misplaced nearly everything I owned. One morning in particular, I raced around the house like a maniac, upending cushions and dumping out the contents of my purse trying to find my missing sunglasses. A few minutes later, my daughter Julie found them in the freezer, lenses frosted over, alongside a church bulletin that I'd used to fan myself during my previous night's power surge.

As I watched my insolent offspring dissolve into a puddle of laughter, I grimly recalled doing the same thing to my own mother twenty-five years earlier, proof positive that what goes around eventually does come back to bite us.

It was time to get practical and make peace with my body. So I picked up the phone and called Mom, the one person who always knew what to do when my head wasn't screwed on straight.

When we sat down to talk face-to-face, I was half expecting an, "I-told-you-so" speech as comeuppance for the bratty way I'd razzed her as she suffered through the change. Heaven knows I deserved it. But instead, she was the essence of comfort and understanding. Then, the strangest thing happened. It was as though a veil suddenly lifted from my eyes, allowing me to observe my own mother for the very first time.

I was startled by her beauty. Her calico eyes with their cool blues, warm browns, and flecks of amber twinkled with humor. Her wavy ash-blonde hair was as thick and full as the day she married my father nearly fifty years earlier. Her elegant poise, confident laugh, and sweet, sparkling smile offered further evidence that Mom was not only one heck of an amazing woman, but her generation's poster child for graceful maturity. And to think I am a part of her gene pool!

I've heard it said that our greatest fear is of the unknown. I was so busy moaning and groaning about the onset of middle age that I never bothered to look at the possibilities. The Big M, with its hot flashes and dwindling hormones, was part of a refining process, preparing me for the chance to emerge from the fire as a more vibrant lady, like my lovely mother.

Many people who see us together remark about how much we're alike. If that's true, I am one very blessed daughter indeed.

Michelle Close Mills

Weeds in My Garden

If we don't change, we don't grow. If we don't grow, we aren't really living.

Gail Sheehy

I stared at my garden on an early fall day, stunned by its overgrown weedy appearance. My thoughts drifted to springtime when I planted the cool, moist soil and watched with anticipation as new life emerged, tender green stems and pastel-colored buds. In the bright and warm summer, the colors and smells of my garden became vibrant and provided a harvest for the senses. Now, as the days cooled, and the thrill of my new garden faded with the summer colors, it occurred to me that I too was in the autumn of my life. This change of season had brought its own weeds to my days and nights such as hot flashes, night sweats, irritability, memory lapses, and sleepless nights.

I knelt in the soil with stiff, achy joints, gloved hands ready to battle the ugly, ragged plants that had invaded my plot. I do love this time of year when the air becomes crisp and the nagging sounds of cicadas have disappeared, leaving only the quiet chirping of birds and crickets. I grabbed hold of the first pesky weed, pulled it, and tossed it over to a small pile. I assailed the demons of my garden for several moments before I looked around and felt overwhelmed by the task at hand. I wanted my garden to be clean and fresh again, without autumn's unattractive overgrowth. I closed my eyes and inhaled the cool air. In my fresh meditative state, I heard wind chimes tinkling in the distance, while all around me I smelled lingering herbs. My mantra began: *One weed at a time, one weed at a time, one weed at a time.*

As I crawled along the ground, I slowly made my way down each formless row. My weed pile became bigger and bigger, assurance that I may yet win the battle. I continued to compare the garden and autumn to this stage in my life and saw the irritating, uncomfortable, sometimes ugly symptoms of menopause as weeds. They too are thorny and unwanted and at times threaten to overtake my life, like my flower garden. I smiled inside as I recognized the weeds of menopause must also be controlled, one weed at a time.

I came upon the green pointed leaves of an iris, its purple bloom of summer long dried and faded. I remembered watching my grandmother in her garden of irises, roses, zinnias, and daisies. Every morning and evening she bent over to pull a weed here, pull a weed there. The fresh flowers she kept on her kitchen table through the spring and summer always added brightness to the conversations that took place over coffee each morning.

Although I loved Grandma's flower patch, as a child I never really understood how she could spend so much time pulling weeds. Now I smiled as I realized Grandma's good, full life was as filled with rich, multicolored blooms as was her garden. And like her garden, her life was not free of its ugly or unpleasant pieces, yet she kept those weeds under control, choosing instead to be thankful for the flowers in her life. When Grandma died, family members harvested seeds and bulbs from her garden and planted them in their own gardens. I looked forward to seeing the purple blooms of Grandma's irises every summer.

One weed at a time, the mound of defeated weeds grew, and the flowers remaining in the garden came back into focus. My garden was filled with brilliant yellow marigolds—my marriage; purple and pink impatiens—my son and daughter; crisp red begonias—my health.

Spring and summer may have passed, but in my garden, still full of lovely flowers, it's a matter of pulling one weed at a time.

Jan Morrill

Supporting Others

The coauthors of *Chicken Soup for the Soul in Menopause* have selected The LifeSkills Center for Leadership, based in Minneapolis, Minnesota, to receive a portion of the book's proceeds.

Character. Confidence. Choice. These are the core beliefs of The LifeSkills Center for Leadership. A nonprofit founded in 2001 by "Famous" Dave Anderson, the organization's objective is to empower youth to believe in themselves, instill a sense of passion and hope, and to strive for their goals and dreams.

The LifeSkills Center for Leadership has been delivering life-changing training to build positive, responsible, and powerful leaders of today and for tomorrow. Upon completion of each training, youth begin the journey of looking at life's challenges as an opportunity to grow, and ultimately become the person they were meant to be.

To learn more, please visit:

The LifeSkills Center for Leadership
1508 East Franklin Avenue, Suite 200
Minneapolis, MN 55404
phone: 612-871-3883
Web site: www.lifeskills-center.org
Web site: www.pathtogreatness.com

Who Is Jack Canfield?

Jack Canfield is the cocreator and editor of the Chicken Soup for the Soul series, which *Time* magazine has called "the publishing phenomenon of the decade." The series includes more than 140 titles with over 100 million copies in print in forty-seven languages. Jack is also the coauthor of eight other bestselling books, including *The Success Principles™: How to Get from Where You Are to Where You Want to Be, Dare to Win, The Aladdin Factor, You've Got to Read This Book,* and *The Power of Focus: How to Hit Your Business, Personal and Financial Targets with Absolute Certainty.*

Jack has recently developed a telephone coaching program and an online coaching program based on his most recent book, *The Success Principles.* He also offers a seven-day Breakthrough to Success seminar every summer, which attracts 400 people from about fifteen countries around the world.

Jack is the CEO of Chicken Soup for the Soul Enterprises and the Canfield Training Group in Santa Barbara, California, and is founder of the Foundation for Self-Esteem in Culver City, California. He has conducted intensive personal and professional development seminars on the principles of success for more than a million people in twenty-nine countries around the world. Jack is a dynamic keynote speaker, and he has spoken to hundreds of thousands of others at more than 1,000 corporations, universities, professional conferences, and conventions and has been seen by millions more on national television shows such as *Oprah, Montel, The Today Show, Larry King Live, Fox and Friends, Inside Edition, Hard Copy, CNN's Talk Back Live, 20/20, Eye to Eye,* and the *NBC Nightly News* and the *CBS Evening News.* Jack was also a featured teacher in the hit movie *The Secret.*

Jack is the recipient of many awards and honors, including three honorary doctorates and a Guinness World Records Certificate for having seven books from the Chicken Soup for the Soul series appearing on the *New York Times* bestseller list on May 24, 1998.

To write to Jack or for inquiries about Jack as a speaker, his coaching programs, trainings, or seminars, use the following contact information:

Jack Canfield
The Canfield Companies
P.O. Box 30880 • Santa Barbara, CA 93130
phone: 805-563-2935 • fax: 805-563-2945
E-mail: info4jack@jackcanfield.com
www.jackcanfield.com

Who Is Mark Victor Hansen?

In the area of human potential, no one is more respected than Mark Victor Hansen. For more than thirty years, Mark has focused solely on helping people from all walks of life reshape their personal vision of what's possible. His powerful messages of possibility, opportunity, and action have created powerful change in thousands of organizations and millions of individuals worldwide.

He is a sought-after keynote speaker, bestselling author, and marketing maven. Mark's credentials include a lifetime of entrepreneurial success and an extensive academic background. He is a prolific writer with many bestselling books, such as *The One-Minute Millionaire, Cracking the Millionaire Code, How to Make the Rest of Your Life the Best of Your Life, The Power of Focus, The Aladdin Factor,* and *Dare to Win,* in addition to the Chicken Soup for the Soul series. Mark has made a profound influence through his library of audios, videos, and articles in the areas of big thinking, sales achievement, wealth building, publishing success, and personal and professional development.

Mark is the founder of the MEGA Seminar Series. MEGA Book Marketing University and Building Your MEGA Speaking Empire are annual conferences where Mark coaches and teaches new and aspiring authors, speakers, and experts on building lucrative publishing and speaking careers. Other MEGA events include MEGA Info-Marketing and My MEGA Life.

As a philanthropist and humanitarian, Mark works tirelessly for organizations such as Habitat for Humanity, American Red Cross, March of Dimes, Childhelp USA, and many others. He is the recipient of numerous awards that honor his entrepreneurial spirit, philanthropic heart, and business acumen. He is a lifetime member of the Horatio Alger Association of Distinguished Americans, an organization that honored Mark with the prestigious Horatio Alger Award for his extraordinary life achievements.

Mark Victor Hansen is an enthusiastic crusader of what's possible and is driven to make the world a better place.

Mark Victor Hansen & Associates, Inc.
P.O. Box 7665 • Newport Beach, CA 92658
phone: 949-764-2640 • fax: 949-722-6912
www.markvictorhansen.com

Who Is Dahlynn McKowen?

Dahlynn McKowen is one of Chicken Soup for the Soul's most trusted and active coauthors. She, along with her husband Ken, coauthored *Chicken Soup for the Fisherman's Soul* (May 2004), and Dahlynn released *Chicken Soup for the Entrepreneur's Soul* in September 2006. The McKowens are currently creating a twelve-book travel series for Chicken Soup for the Soul Enterprises and Health Communications, Inc., a first for both companies, and are coauthoring many more Chicken Soup titles, including *Chicken Soup for the Soul Celebrating Brothers & Sisters* and *Chicken Soup for the Female Entrepreneur's Soul.*

The McKowens stay active with their company Publishing Syndicate, a small business that provides writing, ghostwriting, and editing services to publishers. They also offer a free monthly writing tips e-newsletter and have created an e-booklet series entitled "The Wow Principles." This series, which is sold via their website, focuses on the aspects of writing for publication and profit. The McKowens also author other books each year, the most recent being *Best of California's Missions, Mansions and Museums: Bringing the Golden State's Past Alive for Today's Travelers* for Wilderness Press.

Dahlynn is an established freelance writer with numerous book contracts and screenplays under production at any given moment. Since selling her first feature article in 1987, she has produced more than 2,000 works including business features, B&B reviews, restaurant reviews, and travel articles. Her reputation is such that she has also ghostwritten stories for a former U.S. president, more than two dozen Fortune 100 and 500 corporate founders and CEOs, as well as a few California governors.

Dahlynn loves spending time with her ten-year-old son Shawn and teenage daughter Lahre, who are both active in the family business (a professional photographer and Chicken Soup cartoonist, respectively). She also loves discovering new travel destinations with hubby Ken. Needless to say, her life is not dull by any stretch of the imagination!

Dahlynn McKowen
Publishing Syndicate
P.O. Box 607
Orangevale, CA 95662
www.PublishingSyndicate.com

Contributors

Several of the stories in this book were taken from previously published sources, such as books, magazines, and newspapers. These sources are acknowledged in the permissions section. If you would like to contact any of the contributors for information about their writing or would like to invite them to speak in your community, look for their contact information included in their biographies.

The remainder of the stories were submitted by readers of our previous *Chicken Soup for the Soul* books who responded to our requests for stories. We have also included information about them.

Karen Alexander writes and performs children's poetry and mid-life limericks. Recently, Karen began writing family stories, inspired by her family's move to New Mexico and her new status as "Grandma!" Visit her website at www.abcpoet-tree or e-mail Karen at karenalexander @abcpoet-tree.com.

Judy Quick Anderson lives in a suburb of Minneapolis with her husband and two daughters. Currently at work on a devotional book for the elderly and the dying, Judy also writes devotions for her church community, teaches classes on spiritual gifts, and works one-on-one with those in crisis. E-mail her at vanandjudy@comcast.com.

Nancy Bennett lives on Vancouver Island with her husband, family, and assorted pets. She has been published in more than 300 publications, including *Chicken Soup for the Sister's Soul* and *Tesseracts Ten*. She writes poems, history, and personal essays, as well as dabbles in science fiction.

Genevra Bonati lives in Colorado and loves to play tennis and golf and fly fish with her husband of twenty-seven years, John. The mother of three children, Genevra will embark in the near future into the wonderful world of menopause along with her fellow baby boomers.

Sallie Brown received a bachelor of arts degree in literature from the University of Utah and master of arts degree in counseling and education from the University of Oregon. She taught high school for twenty-seven years. Sallie enjoys writing, walking with her Labrador, driving her Corvette, and quilting. E-mail her at salliebrown@proaxis.com.

Barbara Elliott Carpenter has authored two novels: *Starlight, Starbright* and *Wish I May, Wish I Might,* both available online and in bookstores. Her work appears in national magazines and international websites.

Barbara's interests include painting, quilting, and music. The Carpenters have two children and four grandchildren. E-mail her at bjlogger2@aol.com.

Shae Cooke, a Canadian inspirational writer, mother, and former foster child, shares her heart and God's message of hope internationally. You can learn more about her at http://www.bcfdf.com/thewriters/shaecooke/home.html, contact her at P.O. Box 78006, Port Coquitlam, B.C., Canada V3B 7H5, or e-mail shaesy2000@yahoo.com.

Harriet Cooper is a freelance humorist and essayist living in Toronto, Canada. Her humor, essays, articles, short stories, and poetry have appeared in newspapers, magazines, websites, newsletters, anthologies, radio, and a coffee can. She specializes in writing about family, relationships, cats, psychology, and health.

Cinda Crawford writes suspense/thriller novels. Her latest nonfiction work *From the Floor Looking Up* is a memoir/inspirational health book detailing how she healed from chronic fatigue syndrome, fibromyalgia, and other illnesses. Cinda's life-changing story offers hope and help to millions of people. Website: www.cindacrawford.com.

Vicky DeCoster is an award-winning humor writer and author of *Husbands, Hot Flashes, and All That Hullabaloo!* and *The Wacky World of Womanhood: Essays on Girlhood, Dating, Motherhood, and the Loss of Matching Underwear*. Her work has been published in over sixty magazines and on several websites. Visit www.wackywomanhood.com.

Terri Duncan received her bachelor's, master's, and specialist degrees in education from Augusta State University. She is currently a graduation coach in Evans, Georgia, and is also a devoted wife and the mother of two delightful teenagers. Terri's dream is to publish a full-length book for children.

Lawrence D. Elliott is a nationally published author and has been an active realtor in Southern California since 1989. Along with his wife, Lisa, and dog, Lacie, he lives in Ontario. Lawrence also runs a network of real estate websites, accessible through his main site at www.LawrenceElliott.com.

Earl Engleman has been a cartoonist for thirty-five years. His work has been published in most major publications in the United States and syndicated worldwide through King Features and Singer Media Corp. He can be reached at 352-237-7574.

Judy Epstein, the author of an award-winning humor column, spent almost twenty years prior in public and commercial television, working on everything from documentaries to pledge breaks. But her toughest job, by far, has been just keeping up with her two children.

Sally Friedman, a graduate of the University of Pennsylvania, began her writing career when her youngest started kindergarten. That "child" is now forty. Sally writes about life's cycles—about her own joys and disappointments—and about all the sounds of life. E-mail her at pinegander@aol.com.

Mary Jo Fullhart writes in her spare time when not working with the disabled. She has been published in *Woman's World* and has won an honorable mention in a *Writer's Digest* contest. Her book *Life Of A Leaf* will be released in 2007.

Karen Gaebelein enjoyed a long and rewarding career in the Credit Union industry and has recently retired. While she is looking into other career options, she enjoys writing about everyday topics with a sense of humor to engage her readers and make them laugh. Karen can be reached at gabe501@aol.com.

Ralph Gregory is a graduate of the School of Visual Arts. He has done fine arts, but his passion is creating cartoons and humorous illustrations. Ralph works out at the gym and enjoys listening to music while drawing cartoons in his home studio in Austin, Texas. E-mail him at rgregory5@yahoo.com.

Marilyn Haight lives in Arizona with her husband, Arnold, and their Italian Greyhound, Cameo (aka Sleeping Beauty). When she's not writing "how-to" books, she's searching her soul for stories to craft into personal essays and poetry, hoping to bring more smiles into the world. Website: www.marilynhaight.com.

Janet Hall is a writer, performer, and director. She has published many stories in several publications including numerous stories for the Chicken Soup for the Soul series. You can e-mail Janet at acting-janet@hotmail.com.

Jonny Hawkins is a full-time freelance cartoonist from Sherwood, Michigan. Thousands of his cartoons have appeared in magazines, books and on-line. His calendars, *Medical Cartoon-A-Day* and *Fishing Cartoon-A-Day* can be found online and in bookstores, along with several of his books.

Kim A. Hoyo is a 1974 graduate of the University of Miami, Florida. She recently left south Florida and a successful career as a certified paralegal to move to rural northern Maine and pursue a full-time writing career. You may contact her at kimhoyo@adelphia.net.

Caroleah Johnson has been a practicing dental hygienist for thirty-four years. She and her husband live in the northern California mountains where she bakes bread in a wood-fired oven, relishes grandchildren visits, and pursues her writing passion with the intent of publishing inspirational material. Please e-mail her at caroleah@gmail.com.

Cliff Johnson spent thirty years in prison—in uniform and administration—

and was finally released (retired) in 1995. He enjoys golf, distance running, biking, gardening, metal sculpture, and above all else, his wife Scharre. They live in Crescent City, California, the most beautiful place on earth.

Sally Kelly-Engeman is a freelance writer who's had numerous short stories and articles published. In addition to reading, researching, and writing, she enjoys ballroom dancing and traveling with her husband. She can be reached at sallyfk@juno.com.

Louise Kelman wrote the poem "The Hormone Patch" for her book *Big Purple Undies*. Originally from Birmingham, England, she now lives in Perth, Western Australia and flies all over the world to perform her clean ladies comedy show called "Big Purple Undies." Website: www.bigpurpleundies.com.

Ginger Kenchel is the queen of the Rolla Red Hot Tamales in Missouri, a chapter of the Red Hat Society. A comic at heart, when asked how she stays looking so young, she replies, "Lady Clairol and Oil of Olay, they make me the woman I am today."

Michele H. Lacina received her B.A. in communications from Rowan University in 1973. She began writing in 1999 and has been published in *Country Woman, The Girl's Book of Success* and the *Philadelphia Inquirer*. Michele enjoys music, reading, and travel. She is currently working on a Christian cozy mystery.

Sherri Langton is associate editor of the *Bible Advocate* magazine and *Now What?* e-zine. Her writing has appeared in many Christian publications and several collections, including *Teatime Stories for Women, Becoming a Godly Man,* and *Faces of Faith*. Sherri enjoys walking, swimming, and playing drums and percussion.

Marianne LaValle-Vincent is a published author, poet, and humorist. She has achieved worldwide publication and is currently working as an administrative RN. She lives with her husband, Tim, and sixteen-year-old daughter, Jess. Her entire Italian family gathers at her home each Sunday for dinner. E-mail her at Lavs4@hotmail.com.

Linda Leary began writing in earnest at premenopause and just kept going to postmemopause. Her writing includes articles for local magazines, poetry, editing, web texting, and short stories. In between writing, she enjoys the outdoors and a part-time massage practice. E-mail her at siouxlu@comcast.net.

Patricia Lorenz, the author of seven books, is a top contributor to the Chicken Soup for the Soul series with stories in more than thirty Chicken Soup books. Patricia lives in Florida where she's following her dreams while she's still awake. To hire her as a speaker, e-mail her at patricialorenz@juno.com.

Lorraine Mace is a columnist living in France. Extensively published in the United Kingdom, the United States, Ireland, and France, she has written three children's novels and is the author of e-books *Top Tips to Write for Children* and *Top Tips to Cope Better with Menopause.* Visit her at www.toptipsto.com.

Glady Martin used to write just for her own personal use, but she soon came to see how she was able to express herself openly to others through writing. Her philosphy is that life is an amazing adventure when expressed through words of laughter. E-mail her at gladymartin320@hotmail.com.

Sylvia McClain received her bachelor of general studies in 1999 and is currently working on her master's degree in English. She is a freelance writer for various magazines and teaches workshops in adult education programs. She plans to start writing children's stories. Please e-mail her at sylmcclain@juno.com.

Jacqueline (Jacki) Michels is a mother of five, the wife of one, and a friend to many. She is a columnist and the author of several yet-to-be-published children's stories. Please contact her at jjoila@hotmail.com.

Michelle Close Mills' work has appeared in many magazines, as well as *Chicken Soup for the Recovering Soul Daily Inspirations, The Rocking Chair Reader* and *To Have and To Hold: Prayers, Poems, and Blessings for Newlyweds,* published by Time Warner's Center Street Books. More information: www.authorsden.com/michelleclosemills.

Eileen Mitchell is an award-winning writer who placed second in the 2006 Will Rogers Writing Contest sponsored by the National Society of Newspaper Columnists and 2006 finalist in the Canadian "Writing Fairy" contest. Her essays are published in the book *America's Funniest Humor* and online at HumorPress.com. Blog: MaggiethecatMolly thechihuahua.blogspot.com.

Jan Morrill is pursuing her love of writing after raising two children and spending twenty-five years in the corporate world. She has written several short stories and is working on a novel. When not traveling or sailing, she lives with her husband on a lavender farm in Fayetteville, Arkansas. Contact her at janmorrill@sbcglobal.net.

Rachel S. Neal is a physical therapist enjoying the pristine beauty of western Montana. She writes to inspire, to amuse, and to share the joy of living for Jesus.

Pat Nelson published the book *You—the Credit Union Member* in 1976. She's had careers as a credit union marketing director, a restaurant owner, and a bookkeeper. Now that she's retired, she's enjoying her favorite career—nonfiction writing. Her current project is a book about a former tuberculosis sanatorium.

Bonnie Nester worked for many years as a purchasing agent and is now retired, living on a small farm. She enjoys gardening, horseback riding, and traveling, having just returned from New Zealand and Australia. Bonnie's writing interests are diverse, with Alzheimer's disease being one current subject. Contact: thenester@msn.com.

Lisa Newkirk received her bachelor of arts degree from the University of Denver in 1983. She teaches preschool in Colorado. She enjoys reading, writing, and camping with her family. Please e-mail her at LNewk29762@aol.com.

Brenda Nixon is a professional speaker, writer, and educator for parents. She's the author of *Parenting Power in the Early Years,* and a contributing author to twenty books. She lives in Ohio with her darling husband of twenty-eight years. E-mail: www.brendanixon.com.

Jeanne Pallos is the author of several published articles for adults and children. She is a board member of the Orange County Christian Writers Fellowship in Southern California. Jeanne lives in Laguna Niguel, California, with her husband, Andrew. They are the proud parents of two adult children.

Valerie J. Palmer was born and educated in England but emigrated to Canada in the late 1950s as a teacher. She enjoys nature, reading, art work, print-making, writing poetry, photography, and traveling. She is now retired and lives with her husband, Don, on a farm in Peace River, Alberta.

Connie Parish joined her local Curves nine years ago and was so excited about the concept that she went to work for the company. She became Curves' first area director, owns her own club, and now serves as the area director for South East Texas and Lousiana.

Mark Parisi's "off the mark" comic panel has been syndicated since 1987 and is distributed by United Media. Mark's humor also graces greeting cards, T-shirts, calendars, magazines, newsletters, and books. His wife/business partner, Lynn, and their daughter, Jen, contributes with inspiration (as do three cats). Visit www.offthemark.com.

Ava Pennington is a freelance writer, Bible teacher, public speaker, and former human resources director. She has an MBA from St. John's University, and a bible studies certificate from Moody Bible Institute. She has published magazine articles as well as stories in six Chicken books and other anthologies. E-Mail her at rusavapen@yahoo.com.

Tommy Polk is an award-winning songwriter living in Nashville, Tennessee, and Clarksdale, Mississippi, where he is owner of the Big Pink Guesthouse and part owner of the Shack Up Inn. Websites: www.bigpinkguesthouse.com and www.shackupinn.com.

Valerie Porter has been a freelance writer for more than twenty-five years, specializing in travel, animals, and spirituality. These are also her major interests, so she feels she's been truly blessed. She lives in California with her family and pets and can be reached at vporter27@msn.com.

Linda H. Puckett lives and works with her husband in Arlington, Texas, but her heart belongs to Kentucky. She'll be back home and near her married children when she moves into a national historic home in Greensburg, Kentucky that she and her husband have been remodeling the past two years. Please e-mail her at lhp@hotmail.com.

Robert C. Raina studied art at the University of Massachusetts at Amherst. He is a cartoonist and has written and illustrated several books for children. Robert is the president and owner of a full time entertainment company located in Western Massachusetts. E-mail him at robertraina@cox.net. Websites: bobrainadj.com and bobrainawriting.com.

Joe Rector is a high-school English teacher and freelance columnist. He writes for three newspapers in Knoxville, Tennessee, and has written features for *Sweets Magazine*. Future endeavors include finding a publisher for his book of columns and starting a new magazine for teachers. E-mail him at joerector@comcast.net.

Kathy Reed is a former teacher who lives in Decatur, Alabama. Her stories have been featured in several anthologies, and she was the *Chicken Soup for the Soul Magazine*'s Father's Day story contest winner in 2006. She enjoys travel and playing the mountain dulcimer. Her website is www.writingsbykathy.com.

Terri Reinhardt, married twenty-nine years, has two children and five grandchildren. She is the Queen Mum of her local chapter of the Red Hat Society. She enjoys spending time with her family, especially cooking with her grandchildren, reading, and creative writing. Please e-mail her at thardt27@msn.com.

Donna Rogers is a writer, speaker, and renewal mentor. She wrote *The Menopause Survival Guide*, edits *Midlife Monthly e-Newsletter*, and is a Chicken Soup contributor. She is also the founder of JourneyTo Renewal.org and writes Christian devotionals. Donna enjoys family, friends and e-mails from readers. Website: www.DonnaRogers.com

Joyce Newman Scott worked as a flight attendant for Eastern Airlines while pursuing an acting career. She started college in her mid-fifties, studies at the University of Miami, and is currently working on a memoir, a television script, and a feature film. Please contact Joyce via e-mail at jnewmansco@aol.com.

Jacqueline Seewald earned two graduate degrees from Rutgers University, taught English at the middle school, high school, and college levels and has also worked as an academic librarian and educational media specialist. She has published six fiction books, as well as many short stories, poems, essays, reviews, and articles.

Lahre Shiflet's cartoons have been featured in five Chicken Soup books. Besides drawing, she also likes to sing, model, and act, as well as write original music on her Mac computer to perform. A teenager, hanging out with her friends is Lahre's favorite thing to do!

Dayle Allen Shockley's byline has appeared in dozens of publications. She is the author of three books and has contributed to many other works, including *Chicken Soup for the Sister's Soul 2*. For more information about Dayle, visit www.dayleshockley.com.

Debra Simon, a mar-com professional, received her BA in creative writing. An accomplished musician, Debby also enjoys traveling, hiking, volunteering, and spending time with her family. Her articles have appeared in *The Kansas City Star, STAR* magazine and the anthology *The Kid Turned Out Fine*. Her e-mail address is dksimonsez@sbcglobal.net.

Maggie Lamond Simone, an award-winning writer, is a graduate of William Smith College and S.I. Newhouse School of Communications. Her essays have appeared in *Misadventures of Moms and Disasters of Dads, Hello, Goodbye,* as well as *Cosmopolitan*. She has authored two children's books and an upcoming memoir.

Christine M. Smith is the mother of three, grandmother of thirteen, and foster mother to many others. She has been married to her husband James for thirty-eight years and loves to read, write, participate in church activities, and spend time with her family. Please e-mail her at iluvmyfamilyxxx000@yahoo.com

Elizabeth Sowdal is a freelance writer from Oklahoma City. Postmenopausal, but dealing with it, Elizabeth is married to a tolerant man and has four children who understand that discretion really is the better part of valor—sometimes.

Beverly Spooner has written for all ages but best loves writing for kids. She is published in *Chicken Soup for the Preteen Soul* and in *TRUE—Real Stories About God Showing Up in the Lives of Teens*. Bev lives in Illinois with artist-husband Michael Spooner and son Philip. Please e-mail her at spoonwriter@sbcglobal.net.

Joyce Stark lives in northeast Scotland and has recently retired from local government. She is currently writing a book on her travels in the United States, small towns, backroads, and big cities. You can contact her at joric.stark@virgin.net.

Jean Stewart writes and edits from Mission Viejo, California, where she enjoys her postmenopausal years with her high school sweetheart husband, twin daughters, and two grandchildren. Her stories are also in *Chicken Soup for Fathers and Daughters, Horse Lovers II, Life Lessons for Busy Moms, Dieter's Soul* and other anthologies.

Tena Beth Thompson writes about life and shares her experiences with a touch of humor. She left her hometown in Ohio and now resides in Las Vegas, where she works as a freelance writer. Her column, "A Citizen's View," appears in Las Vegas' *West Valley News.*

Albert Van Hoogmoed, a native of Holland, is a horticulturist in Mobile, Alabama. He has a large collection of funny poetry with a "Far Side" twist that he plans to publish. He can be contacted at vanh6@aol.com.

Beverly Walker is a mother and grandmother who loves writing, photography, and making scrapbooks. She is published in *Chicken Soup for the Cat Lover's Soul* and *Angel Cats: Divine Messengers of Comfort* by Allen and Linda Anderson, and has had poetry published in children's magazines.

Barbara Wenger resides in Elkhart, Indiana, with her husband, Ed. She enjoys doing crafts and spending time with her family and pets. Barbara's favorite days find her sitting on the bank of the river behind her home, writing poetry.

Kathy Whirity is a newspaper columnist. She makes her home in Chicago where she shares her life and love with her husband of thirty years, Bill, and their rambunctious retriever, Hannah. They've discovered, with sweet surprise, that being empty nesters means the honeymoon has only just begun—again.

Diane Dean White is a newspaper columnist and freelance writer. She is the author of *Beach Walks* and *Carolina in the Morning.* She and her husband, Stephen, are the parents of three grown children and three grandgals. They reside on the Carolina coast where they enjoy antiquing.

Jane Wiatrek, a retired educator, spent her career first as a teacher and then as an administrator. She now teaches part-time, does private tutoring, and serves on several community committees and boards. Jane and husband, Ben, live in Poth, Texas, and have three grown sons.

Dick Williams is an ordained minister with the United Methodist Church and currently serves in Everett, Pennsylvania. He and his wife, Pam, have been married for thirty-two years and have two children and two grandchildren.

June Williams lives in Brush Prairie, Washington, with Mac, her husband of forty years. She enjoys spending time with her four wonderful grandchildren. June's stories have appeared in various publications, including *Chicken Soup for the Mother's of Preschoolers Soul* and *Recipes for Busy Moms.* E-mail her at june.williams@comcast.net.

Mary Eileen Williams is a counselor, speaker and writer. Her forthcoming book *Aged to Perfection* might best be described as a saucy combination of Erma Bombeck meets Gloria Steinem while conducting brain research, reviewing women's history, and enjoying a few belly laughs at the fun and foibles of aging. Please e-mail her at agedto perfection@comcast.net.

Sherrin Newsome Willis is a retired retailer from Savannah, Georgia. She now lives in Calhoun, Georgia, where she is a member of a local chapter of the Red Hat Society.

Nancy Withers is currently teaching elementary students in Northern California. She enjoys her daily crossword puzzles and Sudoku when she isn't cooking or playing with her five granddaughters. Nancy hopes to write more stories, plays, and poems for children as well as adults.

Ferida Wolff is a contributor to several Chicken Soup books. She is the author of sixteen books for children, including the picture book *Is a Worry Worrying You?* and will soon have a book published in the United Kingdom. Her essays appear in newspapers and magazines. Her website is www.feridawolff.com.

Marjorie Woodall married her high school sweetheart Darrell Robinson on July 8, 2006, at age fifty. They are making their first home in Olympia, Washington, where "every day is a honeymoon." She can be reached at marjoriewoodall@hotmail.com.

Shannon Woodward is a Calvary Chapel pastor's wife, conference and retreat speaker, and author of *Inconceivable: Finding Peace in the Midst of Infertility* and *A Whisper in Winter: Stories of Hearing God's Voice in Every Season of Life.* Visit Shannon at www.shannonwoodward.com or www.windscraps.blogspot.com.

Lisa Wynn has contributed to publications globally, across North America, Canada, and on-line. She owns Artisans Cup Tea Company, Hell on Heelz, and Artisans Press. Find her at www.artisanspress.com or www.artisanscup.com.

Guaranteed
to make you smile!

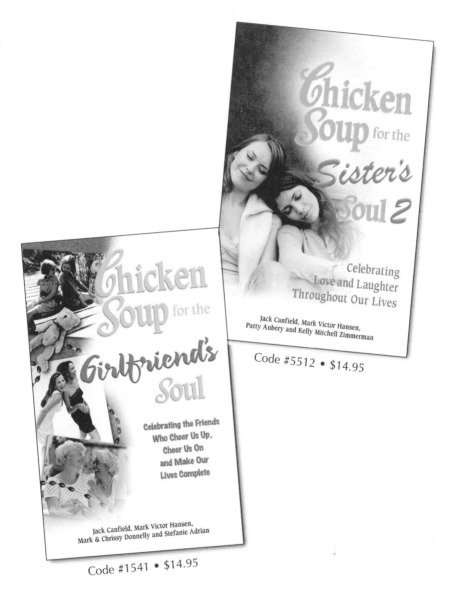

Code #5512 • $14.95

Code #1541 • $14.95